Shamanta Chandran

PHLEBOTOMY
PROCEDURES AND PRACTICES

LYNN B. HOELTKE, M.B.A., M.T. (A.S.C.P.), P.B.T., D.L.M.

❖

DELMAR
CENGAGE Learning™

Australia • Brazil • Japan • Korea • Mexico • Singapore
Spain • United Kingdom • United States

Phlebotomy: Procedures and Practices
Lynn B. Hoeltke

Vice President, Health Care Business Unit:
William Brottmiller

Director of Learning Solutions:
Matthew Kane

Acquisitions Editor: Maureen Rosener

Product Manager: Laurie Traver

Editorial Assistant: Elizabeth Howe

Marketing Director: Jennifer McAvey

Marketing Manager: Christopher Manion

Technology Director: Laurie Davis

Production Director: Carolyn Miller

Production Manager: Barbara A. Bullock

Production Editor: Anne Sherman

© 2006 Delmar, Cengage Learning

ALL RIGHTS RESERVED. No part of this work covered by the copyright herein may be reproduced, transmitted, stored or used in any form or by any means graphic, electronic, or mechanical, including but not limited to photocopying, recording, scanning, digitizing, taping, Web distribution, information networks, or information storage and retrieval systems, except as permitted under Section 107 or 108 of the 1976 United States Copyright Act, without the prior written permission of the publisher.

For product information and technology assistance, contact us at
Cengage Learning Customer & Sales Support, 1-800-354-9706

For permission to use material from this text or product,
submit all requests online at **www.cengage.com/permissions**
Further permissions questions can be emailed to
permissionrequest@cengage.com

Library of Congress Control Number: 2005046641

ISBN-13: 978-1-4180-1054-6

ISBN-10: 1-4180-1054-5

Delmar
Executive Woods
5 Maxwell Drive
Clifton Park, NY 12065
USA

Cengage Learning is a leading provider of customized learning solutions with office locations around the globe, including Singapore, the United Kingdom, Australia, Mexico, Brazil, and Japan. Locate your local office at **www.cengage.com/global**

Cengage Learning products are represented in Canada by Nelson Education, Ltd.

To learn more about Delmar, visit **www.cengage.com/delmar**

Purchase any of our products at your local bookstore or at our preferred online store **www.ichapters.com**

Notice to the Reader
Publisher does not warrant or guarantee any of the products described herein or perform any independent analysis in connection with any of the product information contained herein. Publisher does not assume, and expressly disclaims, any obligation to obtain and include information other than that provided to it by the manufacturer. The reader is expressly warned to consider and adopt all safety precautions that might be indicated by the activities described herein and to avoid all potential hazards. By following the instructions contained herein, the reader willingly assumes all risks in connection with such instructions. The publisher makes no representations or warranties of any kind, including but not limited to, the warranties of fitness for particular purpose or merchantability, nor are any such representations implied with respect to the material set forth herein, and the publisher takes no responsibility with respect to such material. The publisher shall not be liable for any special, consequential, or exemplary damages resulting, in whole or part, from the readers' use of, or reliance upon, this material.

Printed in Canada
5 6 7 8 9 10   13 12 11 10

CONTENTS

List of Procedures   iv

Preface   vii

Learning Objectives   xi

Reviewer Acknowledgments   xv

UNIT 1 ❖ *Venipuncture Principles*   *1*

❖ Focusing on the Patient   1
❖ Customer Service   3
❖ Patient Satisfaction   4
❖ Standard Precautions   5
❖ Blood Components   14
❖ Anticoagulants   18
❖ Why So Many Choices in Types of Tubes   26
❖ Blood Collection Equipment   29
❖ Needle Safety   36
❖ Cleaning of the Draw Site   38
❖ Order of Drawing Tubes   38

UNIT 2 ❖ *Venipuncture Technique*   *41*

❖ Specimen Labeling   41
❖ Test Request Form   46

❖ Precautions in Blood Collection 47
❖ Intravenous Line 49
❖ Vascular Access Device (Line) 50
❖ Handwashing 51
❖ Latex Allergy 51
❖ Collecting the Venipuncture Blood Sample 53
❖ Criteria for Re-collection or Rejection
of a Specimen 86
❖ Factors Affecting Laboratory Values 87
❖ Chilling or Warming of Specimens 90
❖ Blood Cultures 92
❖ Urine Collection 99

UNIT 3 ❖ *Microcollection* 107

❖ Microcollection Equipment 107
❖ Skin Puncture Blood Collection 112
❖ Obtaining a Blood Sample from a
Fingerstick 113

References 121
Appendix A ❖ Phlebotomy Competency Assessment 123
Appendix B ❖ Phlebotomy Test Questions 127
Index 137

List of Procedures

Procedure 1.1 Medical Asepsis Handwashing 7
Procedure 1.2 Removing Contaminated Gloves 11
Procedure 2.1 Proper Patient and Specimen
Identification 41

Procedure 2.2	Tying and Releasing a Tourniquet	57
Procedure 2.3	Venipuncture by Syringe	66
Procedure 2.4	Venipuncture by Evacuated Tube System	73
Procedure 2.5	Venipuncture by Butterfly Needle System	79
Procedure 2.6	Blood Culture Collection	94
Procedure 2.7	Collecting a Cleancatch Midstream Urine Specimen: Male	102
Procedure 2.8	Collecting a Cleancatch Midstream Urine Specimen: Female	103
Procedure 2.9	Collecting a 24-hour Urine Specimen	105
Procedure 3.1	Capillary Blood Collection	116

PREFACE

This handbook on phlebotomy is written to teach phlebotomy skills to individuals who are already familiar with health care. Many individuals working in health care or taking health care–related classes are discovering that they need to have a skill level in phlebotomy. Most phlebotomy textbooks contain information that the health care student or worker is already knowledgeable of. This book keeps it simple by explaining only phlebotomy and the procedures necessary to perform the task. This book is formatted for use in the practicum portion of phlebotomy classes, as the competency and training checklists are ideal for instructors and students to validate that each vital step is performed accurately and competently.

The book is very specific and concise in focusing on adult phlebotomy and specimen collection. It does not attempt to cover anatomy, infant care, or specific laboratory testing such as bleeding times or Unopette procedures. These are left to more complete textbooks, such as *The Complete Textbook of Phlebotomy,* third edition, by this author.

This book is to be used by health care workers needing specific information on phlebotomy procedures. Technical programs in medical assisting or nursing can use this as a supplemental text to teach basic phlebotomy. This book can be covered in several sessions rather than spending an entire semester on the subject. The instructor can use the complementary book, *The Complete Textbook of Phlebotomy,* third edition, and its instructor guide as a resource to answer student questions and develop test questions.

Hospitals and health care institutions that want to update their staff on the basics of phlebotomy can use this book as a reference to the newest and latest procedures and safety devices in use. Multiple pictures accompany procedures, making the learning experience easier. This handbook is an excellent reference guide to use for meeting competency training requirements.

Handbook Organization

This book is organized into three units. Rather than divide the book into chapters, the three units cover the three fundamentals of phlebotomy. The first unit focuses on customer service, the equipment used in phlebotomy, and how this equipment is used. The second unit directs the student in the venipuncture procedure and the variations that exist in obtaining blood. The third unit is dedicated to microcollection of blood.

About the Author

Lynn B. Hoeltke, M.B.A., M.T. (A.S.C.P.), P.B.T., D.L.M., works for a leading joint venture laboratory in the Midwest as laboratory coordinator. He currently teaches phlebotomy as a carrier development program for entry level positions into the laboratory. Lynn has more than 30 years experience in various laboratory leadership roles. He has taught on the technical college level and has developed and taught a nursing-based program for a hospital. He has consulted with several nursing homes and laboratories in teaching phlebotomy techniques to their staff. He has published several magazine articles, been a contributing author for *Comprehensive Medical Assisting,* and is the author of *The Clinical Laboratory Manual Series: Phlebotomy* and *The Complete Textbook of Phlebotomy,* third edition, by Cengage Learning.

LEARNING OBJECTIVES

Unit 1

After studying this unit, the participant will be able to:

1. Describe the manner in which the patient affects the success of the venipuncture.

2. Describe the three different formed elements in the blood.

3. Differentiate between serum and plasma.

4. State the manner in which anticoagulants prevent coagulation.

5. Name the anticoagulant, if any, associated with color-coded tubes.

   a. Gray

   b. Light blue

   c. Lavender

   d. Green

   e. Gold

   f. Red/black

   g. White

6. State the anticoagulant that requires a 1:9 anticoagulant-to-blood ratio and why this is essential.

7. Name the types of tubes that produce a serum specimen.

8. State the purpose of the following additives/tubes:

   a. Serum separation tubes (gel tubes)

   b. Trace element

Unit 2

After studying this unit, the participant will be able to:

1. Explain the implications of not labeling specimens correctly.

2. List all information that must be on the label of a specimen submitted for laboratory testing.

3. State a way to prevent hemoconcentration.

4. List methods to prevent hemolysis during blood collection.

5. Discuss three blood collection alternatives when a patient has an intravenous line running.

6. Describe how much of a discard is pulled from a vascular access device.

7. Explain the single most important way to prevent the spread of infection in a hospital.

8. List four common venipuncture sites.

9. List four techniques that can be used to make a vein easier to feel.

10. State the maximum number of times a venipuncture should be attempted by one person.

11. Explain the importance of proper skin antisepsis in blood culture collection.

12. Explain proper blood culture bottle preparation.

13. Define the following terms:

    a. Cellular elements

    b. Buffy coat

    c. Hemoconcentration

    d. Glycolysis

14. Describe how to successfully perform venipuncture by demonstrating correct:

    a. Selection of equipment

    b. Selection of the appropriate site

    c. Preparation of the site

    d. Venipuncture of the patient

    e. Collection of multiple tubes

    f. Care of the site after collection

15. Indicate the correct order of drawing evacuated tubes and blood culture bottles for venous blood collection.

16. Indicate the three basic methods of collecting a peripheral blood sample.

Unit 3

After studying this unit, the participant will be able to:

1. Describe skin puncture equipment and proper depth of cut for this equipment.

2. Describe the composition of skin puncture blood.

3. Describe what warming of the skin puncture site accomplishes.

4. Determine the safest area of a finger to puncture.

5. Explain the key to an acceptable skin puncture specimen.

6. Explain why hemolysis is more likely in skin puncture blood.

7. State why the first drop of blood is wiped away during skin puncture.

8. Explain the order of draw for microcollection.

REVIEWER ACKNOWLEDGMENTS

Patricia A. Chappell, M.A., B.S.M.T. (A.S.C.P.)
Director, Clinical Laboratory Science
Administrative Director:
Health Science, Medical Assistant
Radiography, Respiratory Therapy, Phlebotomy
Camden County College
Blackwood, New Jersey

Kraig Chugg, M.S., M.T. (A.S.C.P.)
Assistant Professor, Health Sciences
Weber State University
Ogden, Utah

Linda Riipi, Ph.D., M.T. (A.S.C.P.)
Professor and Clinical Education Coordinator
Northern Michigan University
Marquette, Michigan

Julie Stiak, M.E.D., B.S.M.T.
Program Director
Laboratory Assisting and Histology Technician
Phoenix College
Phoenix, Arizona

Christina Thiery, M.L.T. (A.S.C.P.)
Phlebotomy Training Coordinator
Cleveland Clinic Foundation
Cleveland, Ohio

UNIT 1

Venipuncture Principles

Focusing on the Patient

The emphasis in health care is on seeking ways to reduce costs, shorten patient days, and maintain quality care, all while treating the patient as a customer. This customer must be so satisfied with the care that he or she will come back and recommend the health care facility to his or her friends. This is nothing new to health care, but pressures from third-party payers and government regulation have challenged all health care facilities in their ability to cut costs and still satisfy patients. One way to blend these two demands of reducing costs and enhancing patient recognition of care is to use patient-focused care. The most effective method of achieving patient-focused care and reducing costs is to treat the patient as quickly as possible and return that patient to the security and safety of his or her home. The faster the patient can be sent out of the hospital or health care facility, the faster that bed can be refilled with a new patient. For outpatients the same holds true. The faster patients can be serviced, the sooner they can receive appropriate care or diagnosis and the sooner they can return to a normal life. This is the basic economics of any retail store. The more items a store sells in a specific amount of time, the more money that is made. The more patients who come in and out of the health care facility, the stronger the organization is financially.

This type of economics does not negate the needs of the patient. The stronger an organization is financially, the better equipment, specialists, and care the organization can offer the patient. Most patients would rather walk into a modern, clean, and well-maintained building than a building that is in disrepair. The caregiver must keep in mind that each patient is an individual with specific needs. No matter how large the health care organization, when the caregiver is with a patient, that patient should feel that he or she is the only patient that organization is working with that day.

The laboratory plays an integral part in how long it takes the patient to receive proper care. If it takes hours or days to complete necessary testing, the physician is waiting on results and the patient is waiting on treatment. A key delay in result reporting is in the beginning of the testing cycle. This delay is caused by the preanalytical time it takes to obtain the specimen. To speed the process of patient testing, the specimens need to be drawn at the critical moments in that patient's time in the hospital. It takes time to get a phlebotomist up to the nursing unit. The exact moment when that patient should have been tested may have passed. It would be nice to have one phlebotomist for every 10 to 15 patients. That way whenever a specimen needed to be drawn, a phlebotomist would be right there to provide instant phlebotomy. Unfortunately, it would not be cost effective to hire that many phlebotomists. This ratio of patients to phlebotomist can be obtained if the definition of phlebotomist is expanded. As hospitals explore new ways to develop this patient-focused care, the laboratory is often asked to no longer do phlebotomy but to relinquish this duty to the nursing staff.

A mix of reactions from both laboratorians and nurses is seen when this type of shift in duties occurs. The phlebotomy staff is worried about losing their jobs. In addition, there is concern about the quality of the specimens that will be received. The nurses often voice concern because they are being asked to do one more job they do not have time for. These are very valid concerns that need to be addressed before any hospital embarks on the task of using nurses as phlebotomists.

Patient-focused care directs our attention on the patient and what would be best for the patient's comfort. While doing this, the physician and health care facility must get the patient well as rapidly as possible and send the patient home as a satisfied individual.

This book focuses on the methods the phlebotomist can use to make patients' experiences as comfortable and efficient as possible. Patients are generally fearful of having their blood drawn. Surveys of patients often reveal that the procedure patients disliked the most was having their blood drawn. This fear is universal, without reference to who drew the blood.

Communicating with the patient and putting the patient at ease are essential to successful venipuncture. Positive feedback from patients about their experience always stresses how they "did not feel a thing" when their blood was drawn and how the person drawing their blood was "friendly" and "professional." Focusing on the patient during the encounter and communicating with the patient in a friendly, caring manner are keys to compassionate care.

Customer Service

Customer service is composed of many facets that can either make a patient appreciative of quality service or angry because the patient's entire needs were not met. The phlebotomist who meets the patient's needs is the phlebotomist providing the best customer service. Consistently meeting these expectations is difficult.

The phlebotomist works with both external and internal customers. An external customer for the phlebotomist is the patient. But for the phlebotomist, the patient is not the only customer. There are many internal customers, such as the nurse caring for the patient, the physician, the family of the patient, and so on. Each customer has an interest in what the phlebotomist does. The patient wants a caring, pain-free procedure. The physician wants timely, quality results. The family of the patient wants a caring, quality person taking care of the family member. The family also wants someone who keeps them informed and does not treat them as if they are in the way. A simple question to ask is, How would you like to be treated if you were the patient?

To achieve quality service, the phlebotomist must meet three expectations:

1. Know what the customer wants.

2. Determine whether or not the customer is getting the service he or she wants.

3. Continuously take action to satisfy the customer.

Patient Satisfaction

Keeping the patient satisfied is the primary role of the phlebotomist. The customer expects and demands a quality encounter in the phlebotomy experience. The customer will tell other customers that the phlebotomist was excellent at drawing blood, was very friendly, and that the wait was not too long. The patient does not care about the details or the problems of the day; the patient only cares about being treated with compassion and having a quality specimen obtained. Each patient should be treated like a guest in your home. Treat each patient as if he or she is the most important patient of the day, and give that patient individualized attention.

The patient can come into the facility dissatisfied. This is a challenge for the phlebotomist to "read" the customer and improve the customer's satisfaction. Factors affecting the customer's satisfaction

could include a previous negative experience, personality charac-
teristics, high expectations, or the time the patient allowed for the
laboratory visit. If the reality did not match what the patient expected, the patient's experience will be negative. For example, a
negative expectation for the patient is created if the minimum time
it takes for a patient to register and get blood drawn is 15 minutes
but the patient expected the process to be completed in 5 minutes.
For this patient to become satisfied, the patient needs to allow more
time to get his or her blood drawn. Helping the patient understand
the process means taking the time to communicate. The more information the patient is given, the better the patient will understand
how long the process takes. A patient usually is not concerned
about the time if he or she is getting attention during that time.

Standard Precautions

Universal precautions were developed in 1985 by the Centers for
Disease Control and Prevention (CDC) as a response to the increase
in acquired immunodeficiency syndrome (AIDS) and hepatitis B,
both blood-borne diseases. Any patient has the potential to be
infected with these **blood-borne pathogens.** Universal precautions
assume that all blood and most body fluids are potentially infectious. Because it is impossible to know if a patient is infectious, the
health care worker must treat all patients with universal precautions for infection.

Techniques for handling patients' body fluids became known as
body substance isolation (BSI). This required that the health
care worker use gloves whenever handling any type of moist
body substance.

In 1996 the CDC revised universal precautions and released a new
set of guidelines, still in use today, called **standard precautions.**
These precautions create a first tier of precautions for all patients
regardless of their diagnosis or infectious status.

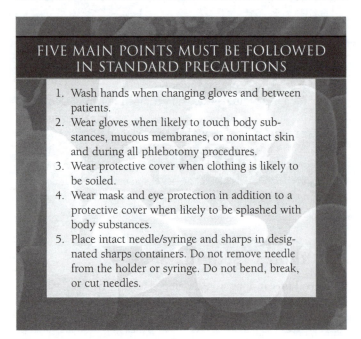

FIVE MAIN POINTS MUST BE FOLLOWED IN STANDARD PRECAUTIONS

1. Wash hands when changing gloves and between patients.
2. Wear gloves when likely to touch body substances, mucous membranes, or nonintact skin and during all phlebotomy procedures.
3. Wear protective cover when clothing is likely to be soiled.
4. Wear mask and eye protection in addition to a protective cover when likely to be splashed with body substances.
5. Place intact needle/syringe and sharps in designated sharps containers. Do not remove needle from the holder or syringe. Do not bend, break, or cut needles.

Handwashing and Disinfecting

Handwashing is a work practice control that is incorporated into the phlebotomist's work habits to prevent the spread of infection. Handwashing is the single most important way to prevent the spread of infection. Hands should be washed under running water with soap and vigorous rubbing.

Handwashing is the method of choice for removing any surface bacteria from the skin. Hands must be washed after removing gloves because the gloves may have defects where contaminants (bacteria or viruses) can penetrate.

Procedure 1.1 illustrates the proper method for medical asepsis handwashing.

Procedure 1.1

MEDICAL ASEPSIS HANDWASHING

Principle:

To clean the hands with the use of soap and running water and reduce the number of organisms on the hands and wrists. The purpose is to decrease the transfer of organisms from a source to a susceptible host.

Materials:

Sink with running water, preferably with foot- or electric eye–operated controls.

Soap from a foot-operated container or pump container.

Disposable paper towels.

Nailstick and/or brush.

Procedure:

1. Remove all rings, watches, and so on to prevent the jewelry from harboring microorganisms.

2. Have disposable towels ready so you do not have to touch the towel dispenser.

3. Stand back from the sink so that you or your clothing does not touch the sink.

4. Turn on the water with the foot pedal or with a disposable towel if not foot controlled. Temperature should be lukewarm (Figure 1.1).

5. Wet hands under the running water. Be careful to not touch the sides of the sink (Figure 1.2).

continues

Procedure 1.1 *continued*

MEDICAL ASEPSIS HANDWASHING

FIGURE 1.1 *Prepare towels for use; turn on water.*

FIGURE 1.2 *Wet hands under running water.*

6. Apply soap, and lather well. The lather and friction scrubbing action will remove dirt and dead skin. Scrub between fingers and around fingernails (Figure 1.3). Use a nailstick and a brush during the first handwashing of each day or when your hands become excessively soiled (Figures 1.4 and 1.5).

7. Rinse hands with the water flowing downward off the fingertips. This will rinse the contaminated water off the fingertips and not onto the forearms (Figure 1.6).

8. Complete the washing process again if this is the first handwashing of the day. (Repeat steps 6 and 7.)

9. Dry hands and wrists with the disposable towels.

10. Turn off water with the disposable towels if the sink is not foot controlled or electronically controlled.

continues

Procedure 1.1 *continued*

MEDICAL ASEPSIS HANDWASHING

FIGURE 1.3 *Apply soap and lather well.*

FIGURE 1.4 *Use a nailstick under fingernails.*

FIGURE 1.5 *Use a brush to clean around fingernails.*

FIGURE 1.6 *Rinse off hands with water flowing downward off hands.*

Antiseptic nonwater hand cleaners or antiseptic towelettes are acceptable in place of handwashing when running water is not available. Antiseptic cleaners have become widely accepted because people are more compliant with the hand cleaner than with washing hands. It is very simple when going from one patient to another to rub hand cleaner into your hands. This takes less time than a proper handwashing. However, nonwater hand cleaners contain alcohol, and prolonged use dries the skin. It is preferable to wash hands with soap and running water if at all possible.

Disinfecting of hard surfaces such as countertops is accomplished with a sterile technique. Disinfecting solutions are too harsh for the skin, but they can kill up to 100 percent of the contaminants. Total sterilization of human skin is not acceptable because the chemicals used are too harsh. Multiple solutions are commercially available for the sterilization of work surfaces. Commercially available solutions usually come in spray bottles or towelette wipes. The least expensive and most effective is 10 percent household bleach. This can be made by adding 1 part bleach to 10 parts water and then either spraying it or wiping it on the surface. Bleach solution must be made daily. Whenever a 10 percent bleach solution is made, the container must be marked with the time and date the solution was made. If it has been more than 24 hours, the solution must be discarded and a new solution made with a new date and time documented on the container.

Gloves

There are three reasons for wearing gloves in patient care:

1. Sterile gloves prevent health care workers from transmitting their own microflora to the patient, such as during surgery or wound cleansing.

2. Gloves prevent the transmission of microorganisms from one patient to another.

3. Gloves prevent the phlebotomist from becoming infected with what is infecting the patient.

Always remove gloves according to Procedure 1.2.

Procedure 1.2

REMOVING CONTAMINATED GLOVES

Principle:

To remove gloves after use to avoid contamination of the phlebotomist. The purpose is to decrease the transfer of organisms from a patient to a phlebotomist or phlebotomist to a patient.

Materials:

Gloves sized to properly fit.

Biohazard waste container.

Procedure:

1. Hold hands out in front of the body.
2. Grasp the palm of one hand, and pull down on the glove to pull the glove inside out. A right-handed person would naturally pull the palm of the left hand (Figures 1.7 to 1.10).
3. The hand still having the glove on should then hold the removed glove (Figure 1.11).
4. Insert two fingers of the ungloved hand under the cuff of the glove of the other hand (Figure 1.12).
5. Pull down on this glove to turn the glove inside out. This will invert the glove and contain the other glove inside the inverted glove (Figures 1.13 and 1.14).
6. Dispose of gloves in a biohazard waste container (Figure 1.15).

continues

Procedure 1.2 *continued*

REMOVING CONTAMINATED GLOVES

FIGURE 1.7 *Grasp the palm of the used glove.*

FIGURE 1.8 *Begin removing the first glove.*

FIGURE 1.9 *Pull down on the glove inside out.*

FIGURE 1.10 *Pull the left glove into the right glove.*

continues

Procedure 1.2 *continued*

REMOVING CONTAMINATED GLOVES

FIGURE 1.11 *Hold the glove in the right hand.*

FIGURE 1.12 *Insert two fingers under the cuff of the other glove.*

FIGURE 1.13 *Use the ungloved fingers to pull the glove inside out.*

FIGURE 1.14 *One glove is now inside the other.*

continues

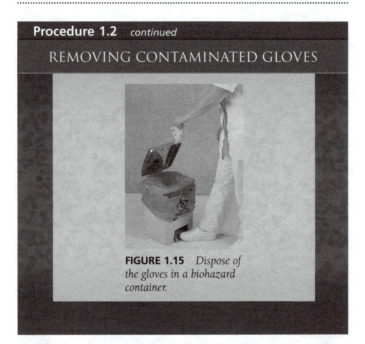

Procedure 1.2 *continued*

REMOVING CONTAMINATED GLOVES

FIGURE 1.15 *Dispose of the gloves in a biohazard container.*

Blood Components

The blood of an adult consists of about 45 percent formed elements. The formed cellular elements are **erythrocytes** (red blood cells), **leukocytes** (white blood cells), and **thrombocytes** (platelets) (Figure 1.16).

Generally, 2 milliliters of blood yields about 1 milliliter of fluid. In the body, the liquid portion is called plasma. When the blood is removed from the body and allowed to clot, the liquid portion is called serum.

Whole blood = plasma
Clotted blood = serum

WBC
(Leukocyte)

RBC
(Erythrocyte)

Platelet
(Thrombocyte)

FIGURE 1.16 *Formed cellular elements of the peripheral blood.*

The clot contains all the formed elements intertwined together in a fibrin mass. Blood flowing through the body contains a substance called fibrinogen. Once the blood leaves the body, the fibrinogen turns into fibrin. This fibrin is like a sticky spider web and traps the formed elements into the fibrin mass called a clot. The clot then contracts, and the liquid (serum) portion is extracted. This serum is a clear straw-colored liquid that is used for many of the tests done in the laboratory.

Different tests require different types of blood specimens. Some specimens require a serum sample. The tube used will be one that allows the blood to clot, such as a red-, gold-, or red/black-stoppered tube. Others require a whole-blood or plasma specimen and need to be drawn in a specimen container that does not allow it to clot. To prevent clotting of the blood, the tube contains an anticoagulant. An anticoagulant is a chemical substance that prevents coagulation by removing calcium and forming calcium salts or by inhibiting the conversion of prothrombin to thrombin. Both calcium and thrombin are part of the coagulation cascade (Figure 1.17). The coagulation cascade is like a staircase in which a ball is bounced down each step. The blood clots when the ball reaches the bottom of the stairs. If a step is taken away, the ball does not reach the bottom of the stairs and the blood does not clot. This staircase contains many steps. These steps

FIGURE 1.17 *Coagulation cascade.*

consist of different chemicals and factors that are required for a person's blood to clot. A person with a bleeding disorder has one of the factors missing or is physically unable to use a needed chemical. One disorder of this type is hemophilia. The patient can temporarily overcome this bleeding disorder by receiving an appropriate factor. A person with hemophilia has one of the steps in the staircase missing. By giving the person with hemophilia a factor such as factor VIII, the step is rebuilt and clotting occurs.

This process of clotting can be stopped in the test tube. A tube containing an anticoagulant removes one of the steps to the staircase, meaning the blood will not clot. The anticoagulant prevents clotting depending on the anticoagulant used. The anticoagulants used are oxalates, citrates, ethylenediaminetetraacetic acid (EDTA), and heparin.

In the process of going down the stairs, five basic steps occur.

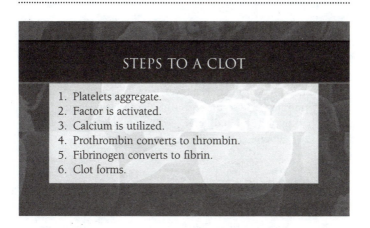

STEPS TO A CLOT

1. Platelets aggregate.
2. Factor is activated.
3. Calcium is utilized.
4. Prothrombin converts to thrombin.
5. Fibrinogen converts to fibrin.
6. Clot forms.

When the blood specimens are centrifuged, a layering of the elements of the blood occurs (Figure 1.18). To produce a plasma specimen, the blood has to be prevented from clotting. In an anticoagulated tube of blood that has been centrifuged, the formed elements and plasma are layered according to weight. The bottom

FIGURE 1.18 *Blood tubes.*

layer contains erythrocytes; then there is a thin layer called the buffy coat, which contains a mixture of leukocytes and thrombocytes. On top of these layers is the plasma layer. The plasma contains fibrinogen and usually is slightly hazy. To produce a serum specimen, the blood must be allowed to clot. This usually takes at least 15 minutes. The serum forms on the top layer, with the clot on the bottom. The main difference between serum and plasma is that plasma contains fibrinogen and serum does not.

Anticoagulants

Anticoagulants work on two principles. The anticoagulant either precipitates/removes the calcium or stops the prothrombin-to-thrombin reaction from progressing. A variety of tubes are available with different anticoagulants for various laboratory testing. The most common tube types are listed in Figure 1.19.

Gray-stoppered Tubes

Gray-stoppered tubes contain potassium oxalate in combination with another weak anticoagulant, sodium fluoride. The anticoagulant combination of potassium oxalate and sodium fluoride works by precipitating out the calcium in the blood and therefore stopping the coagulation cascade. The fluoride's primary function is not as an anticoagulant but as a glycolytic inhibitor. The fluoride preserves the glucose in the blood sample by inhibiting the enzymes involved in breakdown of the glucose (glycolysis). As a blood sample sits without the fluoride, the glucose is broken down at a rate of around 7 percent per hour. A sample that was drawn from a patient and left to sit will have a falsely lower glucose value. This can be pictured as little men opening their mouths and devouring the glucose molecules. Over time there would be no glucose molecules left. The fluoride keeps these men from opening their mouths and helps preserve the glucose.

Tube Color	Additive	Additive Action	Laboratory Use	Laboratory Department
Gray	Potassium oxalate/sodium fluoride or sodium fluoride/EDTA	Binds calcium/ stabilizesglucose values	Glucose testing	Chemistry
Light Blue	Sodium citrate	Binds calcium	Use for coagulation studies. Tubes must be filled to the proper level.	Coagulation
Lavender	Ethylene diaminetetra - acetic acid (EDTA)	Binds calcium	Hematology testing	Hematology
Green	Lithium heparin or sodium heparin	Inhibits Prothrombin to thrombin formation	Plasma determinations in chemistry.	Stat chemistry
Royal Blue	Sodium heparin, EDTA or no additive	Inhibits thrombin formation, binds calcium or clots	Plasma or serum toxicology	Special heavy metals testing
Red	Glass tube – no additive Plastic tube – clot activators	Clot forms	Serum for various tests	Blood Bank, Immunology, Drug testing
SST, Gold or Red/ Black	Clot activators, gel separator	Clot forms	Serum for various tests	Chemistry
Orange	Thrombin clot activator	Clot forms	Stat serum testing	Stat Chemistry
Pink	EDTA	Binds calcium	Immuno- hematology testing	Blood Bank

FIGURE 1.19 *Tube guide.*

Often there is a delay between when a sample is drawn from a patient and when it makes it to the laboratory to be tested. What is being monitored is the glucose of that patient at the time the sample was drawn. If the glucose was allowed to decrease in the sample, the results at the time of testing would indicate that the patient had a glucose value less than actual. The patient would then be falsely treated for a low glucose. The way to prevent this is to draw samples to be tested for glucose in a gray-stoppered tube if there is to be a delay in testing. This tube is used for glucose tests such as fasting blood sugar (FBS), random blood glucose, post-prandial glucose, and glucose tolerance tests.

Light Blue–stoppered Tubes

Light blue–stoppered tubes contain the anticoagulant sodium citrate. Sodium citrate prevents the coagulation by binding calcium in a nonionized form. The sodium citrate anticoagulant most widely used is 3.2 percent buffered sodium citrate (0.105M). Citrate is used primarily in coagulation studies. It is critical that the light blue–stoppered tubes be filled to their proper level for accurate patient results. A ratio of one part anticoagulant to nine parts blood must be maintained. If a tube is only half filled, the ratio will be off and the results will be invalid. The anticoagulant in the tube prevents the blood from clotting by binding the calcium. To test the blood for coagulation studies, the blood is centrifuged to produce a plasma specimen. An aliquot of this plasma specimen combines with other chemicals to restart the coagulation process and produce a clot. The time it takes for a visible clot to form is the result for the coagulation study. There are normal time ranges for this clotting to occur, and an abnormal result falls outside these ranges. Tests using the light blue–stoppered tube to detect clotting problems include prothrombin time (PT), activated partial thromboplastin time (aPTT), D-dimer, fibrin split products, factor assays, and fibrinogen assay.

Lavender-stoppered Tubes

Lavender-stoppered tubes contain the anticoagulant EDTA. This anticoagulant also binds the calcium to prevent coagulation. EDTA comes in two forms, either liquid (K3EDTA) or powder (K2EDTA). Liquid EDTA is found in the glass tubes, and powdered EDTA is found in the plastic tubes. EDTA is the anticoagulant of choice for hematology procedures. Dipotassium EDTA is now the anticoagulant for hematology recommended by the International Council for Standardization in Hematology (ICSH) and Clinical and Laboratory Standards Institute. Dipotassium EDTA is recommended because it preserves cell morphology for complete blood cell counts (CBCs) and differential blood smears and provides stable microhematocrit results. Other anticoagulants distort the size and shape of the cells. This distortion often makes it appear that a disease process is occurring in the patient, when it is actually the effects of the anticoagulant. Tests using the lavender-stoppered tube are CBC, hemoglobin (Hgb), hematocrit (Hct), and hemoglobin A_1C.

Green-stoppered Tubes

Up to this point, all the anticoagulants discussed have prevented coagulation by precipitating or binding the calcium in the blood. Green-stoppered tubes contain heparin, which stops coagulation by inhibiting the conversion of prothrombin to thrombin and thus inhibiting the following stages that lead to a clot. What has occurred is that no fibrin is formed to cause a clot. Heparin is a naturally occurring substance that is present in most of our tissues, but at low levels. Because of this it has the least effect on clinical chemistry tests of all the anticoagulants. It produces the least stress on erythrocytes and minimizes hemolysis. This is the anticoagulant of choice for pH determinations, electrolyte studies, and arterial blood gases. The two most commonly used forms of heparin are lithium heparin and sodium heparin. Before drawing a test with a heparin tube, you must know what type of heparin is acceptable. Some tests are affected by the presence of the lithium or sodium. If the lithium or sodium has an effect, then the alternate heparin tube must be used.

Solution A or B

Solution A and solution B yellow-stoppered tubes contain variations of a mixture of trisodium citrate, citric acid, and dextrose. Solution A has a higher concentration than solution B. They are used for DNA and paternity testing, human leukocyte antigen (HLA) phenotyping, and some immunohematology studies.

Sodium Polyanthol Sulfonate

A yellow-stoppered tube that contains acid citrate dextrose (ACD) as an anticoagulant is used for collecting blood culture samples. This yellow-stoppered tube looks the same as the two previously discussed tubes except it contains the additive sodium polyanthol sulfonate (SPS). The yellow-stoppered tubes can be confusing in that there are multiple types of yellow-stoppered tubes with specific uses. The phlebotomist must read the label before using one of these tubes to ensure that the proper tube with the proper additive is used. Blood cultures are also collected using specific aerobic and anaerobic blood culture bottles.

Pink-stoppered Tubes

Pink-stoppered tubes contain the anticoagulant EDTA, which binds the calcium to prevent coagulation and is the same anticoagulant as the K2EDTA in the lavender-stoppered tubes. This tube is made for immunohematology testing and is designed with a special crossmatch label for required information by the American Association of Blood Banks (AABB).

Orange-stoppered Tubes

Thrombin is a clot activator used for STAT (emergency) testing. The thrombin is within the tube to hasten the clotting process faster than silica particles. These tubes usually have an orange stopper. Most chemistry tests that can be performed on serum can use this tube as a substitute.

White-stoppered Tubes

White-stoppered tubes contain EDTA as an anticoagulant and also a gel to separate the plasma from the cells. A specimen for EDTA plasma can be collected in this tube, the tube centrifuged, and then frozen without pouring off the plasma into a separate tube. This is especially helpful in working with human immunodeficiency virus (HIV)– positive patients. Processing the blood without a need to open the tube provides greater safety for the phlebotomist. This tube is used for molecular diagnostic tests such as polymerase chain reaction (PCR) or branched DNA amplification techniques.

Royal Blue–stoppered Tubes

Drawing blood for trace elements is when blood is being tested for heavy metals such as arsenic or lead. The only difference in the collection is that the blood must be collected in a special metal-free tube. These are usually royal blue–stoppered tubes that may or may not contain an anticoagulant. The glass and rubber stoppers have been specially refined to be metal free. Traces of metal in the routinely used evacuated tube may leach into the specimen and give the patient a falsely elevated heavy metal value. The tubes have sodium heparin, EDTA, or no additive and a green, lavender, or red band on the label to indicate the type of additive or no additive in the tube. Therefore the phlebotomist must read the label carefully to verify the type of tube being used.

Glass Red-stoppered Tubes

The glass red-stoppered tube is the traditional tube used when a serum sample from a clotted tube of blood is needed. The glass red-stoppered tube has no anticoagulants. Most blood collection tubes have a silicon coating on the interior surface of the tube. This silicon fills the microscopically rough surface of the glass. Glass may feel smooth to the touch, but it has a rough surface that cells can stick to. The silicon fills these cracks and crevasses and prevents the cells from adhering to the glass surface. This reduces the chance for hemolysis and makes the sides slicker so the cells can centrifuge to the bottom of the tube faster. These tubes have a red stopper, red/black stopper, or gold stopper (Hemogard brand tube), depending on the manufacturer.

Plastic Red-stoppered Tubes

The glass surface of a tube used for serum testing activates clot formation in the tube. Some glass serum tubes have a clot activator added to speed the clotting process. A plastic tube will not activate a clot, and therefore a clot activator must be added to each tube during manufacture of the tube. The clot activator added to the tubes is a silica coating on the sides of the tubes. Various additives are added to the tubes to improve the quality of the specimen. These additives are not anticoagulants or preservatives but are used to improve specimen quality or accelerate specimen processing.

Gel Separator

Serum and plasma tubes can also be purchased with a thixotropic separator gel (Figure 1.20). This gel is an inert material that undergoes a temporary change in viscosity during centrifugation. It has a density that is intermediate to cells/clot and plasma/serum. When centrifuged, the gel moves up the sides of the tube and engulfs the cells/clot; an interface of gel forms that separates the cells/clot from the plasma/serum (Figure 1.21). These tubes are often called SSTs, for serum separator tubes, or PSTs, for plasma separator tubes.

The separator gel helps preserve the constituents of the serum/plasma so that the chemistries being tested for will not deteriorate if testing cannot be done immediately. The gel preserves the serum/plasma without the need to aliquot the serum/plasma into a

FIGURE 1.20 *Separator gel tubes.*

separate plain tube. This provides a savings in extra tubes and makes processing the tube faster and safer. The gel allows the tube to be transported without the cells mixing with the serum/plasma. The gel traps the cells in the bottom of the tube.

Blood Gel	Serum or Plasma Cells Gel	Serum or Plasma Gel Cells	Serum or Plasma Gel Cells
Before Centrifugation	During Centrifugation	Plug Formation	After Centrifugation

FIGURE 1.21 *Separator gel tubes: centrifugation process.*

Why So Many Choices in Types of Tubes

Many choices need to be made to collect the correct sample when drawing blood from a patient. There are many different tubes to select from, and different tests require different tubes. Trying to understand why one tube cannot do all the testing often gets confusing. This was explained to some degree in the section on anticoagulants.

Only two types of tubes are collected from a patient: tubes that clot, and tubes that have an anticoagulant in the tube to prevent clotting. The clotted tube produces liquid serum, and the anticoagulant tube produces liquid plasma. For a tube to clot, the blood in the tube must go through several steps:

1. Platelet clumping (platelet aggregation)
2. Factor activation
3. Calcium present to activate clotting
4. Prothrombin converting to thrombin
5. Fibrinogen converting to fibrin
6. Final clot formation

Blood placed in a red-stoppered tube goes through all these steps. Tubes with gel serum separator (SSTs) go through the same steps. The gel in the tube works to separate the serum from the clot. The gel also has been known to absorb some of the drugs being tested, so it is not used for drug monitoring. Even though both types of tubes produce a serum specimen, they each have their own reason for being collected.

Anticoagulant tubes are collected when nonclotted whole blood or plasma is needed. Each tube is unique in its use in testing, and the anticoagulants work differently. Any blood placed in these tubes will try to go through the clotting process, but the anticoagulant, if properly mixed with the blood, will prevent this from occurring. The methods that the tubes incorporate to prevent the clotting are listed in Figure 1.22.

Tube Type	Anticoagulant	Prevents clotting by:
Lavender stoppered	EDTA	Removing the calcium to stop the coagulation process
Gray stoppered	Potassium oxalate/ Sodium fluoride	Potassium oxalate removes the calcium. Sodium Fluoride preserves the glucose.
Light Blue stoppered	Sodium citrate	Binds the calcium to stop the coagulation
Green stoppered	Either Lithium heparin or Sodium heparin	Stops the prothrombin to thrombin reaction.

FIGURE 1.22 *Methods to prevent clotting in tubes.*

What Figure 1.22 illustrates is that the anticoagulants work in a variety of methods to prevent the blood from clotting. This is why often one type of tube or the plasma/serum from a tube cannot be substituted for another. Some examples of problems that can occur when an incorrect sample is sent include the following:

1. A blood sample is collected in a sodium heparin green-stoppered tube, and the plasma is pulled off to test for a sodium level on the patient. The sodium level of the patient will be falsely elevated due to the sodium in anticoagulant.

2. A blood sample is collected in a gray-stoppered tube and submitted for a CBC. The gray-stoppered tube will not work as a replacement for the lavender-stoppered tube. The EDTA anticoagulant in the lavender-stoppered tube preserves the morphology of the red blood cells and white blood cells. If the gray-stoppered tube is used to determine the CBC results, the cells will appear abnormal and the patient's normal cells could be reported as abnormal.

3. A lavender-stoppered tube is used instead of a clot tube for a calcium test. The person drawing the blood feels no one will notice the mistake and centrifuges the lavender-stoppered tube. The plasma is pulled off and sent to the laboratory. The results indicate that the patient has a zero calcium level. This is a result of the anticoagulant, EDTA, removing the calcium from the plasma to prevent the blood from clotting.

4. A light blue–stoppered tube is used to collect a specimen from the patient, and the phlebotomist notices before taking the needle out of the patient's arm that the tube did not fill completely. A second tube is drawn, and it does not fill completely. To submit a completely filled tube as is required, the two half-filled tubes are poured together. The patient's test result will be incorrect because by pouring the two tubes together, the amount of anticoagulant in the combined tube is doubled.

Unfortunately there is no "one size fits all" in the collection of blood specimens. The testing methods are very specific and require the correct sample type. A specific tube must be used for a specific test. Mixing of blood samples from different tubes or combining two half-filled tubes will alter the patient's results.

Blood Collection Equipment

All blood collection equipment utilizes invasive techniques to open a vein to obtain a sample. The common equipment used today punctures the vein and evacuates the blood sample without destroying the integrity of the vein.

The recommended length of the needle used in venipuncture is 1 to 1½ inches. The gauges of needles used are 25, 23, 22, 21, 20, 18, and 16, with the smallest diameter needle being a 25 gauge and the largest being a 16 gauge.

Needle Gauge	Needle Use
25	Intramuscular injections
23	Butterfly collection system or syringe collection
22	Syringe or evacuated system collection
21	Syringe or evacuated system collection
20	Syringe or evacuated system collection
18	IVs or blood donation
16	IVs or blood donation

The needles come in different gauges for the different size veins that need to be accessed or the amount of blood that needs to be taken. For a child, or an adult when only one tube of blood must be collected, a 23- or 22-gauge needle is appropriate. When someone is donating a unit of blood, the blood needs to be collected faster, so a 16- or 18-gauge needle is used. The needle should be thought of as a pipeline. The faster you want the blood to flow, the larger the pipeline you will need. Consideration must also be made for the size of the vein. The pipeline must fit inside the vein. Therefore the needle must be small enough to fit inside the vein. This size also partially controls the vacuum of the blood pulling on the vein. A large needle with a large evacuated tube produces a large amount of vacuum on the vein and may possibly collapse the vein. A smaller needle paired with a smaller tube reduces the vacuum.

The 25-gauge needle cannot be used for venipuncture because the red blood cells would be destroyed (hemolyzed) when blood is pulled through the bore of the needle. The best alternative is to use a 23-gauge needle with a butterfly collection set. This gives access to small veins but does not result in hemolysis of the cells.

Needle size is the choice of the phlebotomist. The phlebotomist must analyze each situation and determine the best equipment to obtain the blood sample.

All needles for venipuncture are manufactured with an angled bevel on the tip of the needle. This bevel helps the needle enter the skin and reduces the pain upon entry. It also gives a larger opening in the tip of the needle to enhance blood flow.

Syringe System

The syringe and needle method of collecting blood is one of the oldest methods known that does not destroy the integrity of the vein. The principle and basic construction have remained the same: a sleeve with a plunger that fits inside, and a needle attached to the other end. The barrel and plunger vary in volume from 1 milliliter to 60 milliliters. The plunger creates a vacuum within the barrel. The plunger on a syringe often sticks and is hard to pull. A technique called "breathing the syringe" needs to be done before it is used. To breathe the syringe, pull back on the plunger slightly and then push the plunger back. This makes the plunger pull more smoothly and reduces the tendency to jerk when first pulled.

A large syringe collects more blood, but it can also create a problem, producing too much vacuum and collapsing the vein. Pulling the plunger slowly and resting between pulls allows the vein time to refill with blood and prevents collapse of the vein. Generally syringes are used for the difficult-to-draw patients who have fragile, thin, or "rolly" veins. Pediatric or geriatric patients typically have these types of veins. The use of a syringe and needle is limited by the capacity of the syringe. The use of a syringe larger than 10 to 15 milliliters to collect blood from fragile veins is not recommended. If a large amount of blood is needed, a butterfly collection set is to be used. Syringes are also used in special procedures when the blood must be drawn and then transferred to a different container.

For the protection of the phlebotomist, the syringe should have a safety shield that covers the needle incorporated into the device (Figure 1.23).

FIGURE 1.23 *Syringe and needle with safety sleeve for needle.*

Evacuated System

The evacuated system is often called the Vacutainer system. Vacutainer can be a misnomer, because it is a brand name for the evacuated system manufactured by the Becton Dickinson Company.
The Vacutainer name has become synonymous with all evacuated
blood collection systems.

The evacuated blood collection system is a closed system that
adds an element of safety. In the evacuated system, a tube containing a vacuum attaches to the needle and the tube's vacuum is
replaced by blood. The tubes can be glass or plastic (Figure 1.24).
The total system consists of a double-pointed needle, a plastic
holder or adapter, and a series of vacuum tubes with rubber
stoppers. One end of the double-pointed needle enters the
patient, and the opposite end of the needle punctures the stopper
of the tube.

The key to the evacuated system is the double-pointed needle,
with a different length needle on each end and a screw hub near
the center. The longer needle has a bevel that enters the vein. The
shorter needle pierces the rubber stopper in the blood collection

FIGURE 1.24 *Assorted types of evacuated tubes.*

tube. The needle that pierces the rubber stopper of the tube has a sleeve that functions as a valve to stop the flow of blood when the tube is removed. Pushing the tube into the holder compresses the sleeve and exposes the needle as it enters the tube. When removing the tube, the sleeve slides back over the needle and stops the flow of blood. The needle pictured has a safety shield attached to the needle that covers the needle after use (Figure 1.25).

The needle must be thought of as a pipeline that is going to deliver blood from the patient to the tube. The blood is pulled out of the patient due to the vacuum inside the tube.

The patient will experience the least pain if the bevel of the needle is facing upward when inserted into the vein. The bevel of the needle is upward when looking straight down on the needle as the needle is inserted into the skin; the opening in the needle will be visible. The needle should be inserted at a 15-degree angle to the surface of the skin (Figure 1.26). This technique allows the point of the needle to enter the skin first with little

FIGURE 1.25 *Evacuated tube needle with safety shield attached.*

FIGURE 1.26 *Proper angle of insertion.*

dragging or bunching up of the skin and reduces the pain of the puncture.

The holder for the needle makes the task of collecting the blood sample easier. The holders have changed in recent years to include holders with covers that snap closed over the contaminated needle. (Figure 1.27)

Butterfly

A winged infusion set (butterfly) consists of a ¹⁄₂- to ³⁄₄-inch stainless steel needle connected to a 6- to 12-inch length of tubing. It is called a butterfly because of its wing-shaped plastic extensions, which are used for gripping the needle. Butterfly needles for venipuncture are 25, 23, or 21 gauge. A 25-gauge butterfly and syringe should be avoided because an increased chance for hemolysis exists.

Butterflies generally come with ports that allow them to be used with syringes, or with multiple sample Leur adapters, allowing them to be used with an evacuated tube system. Leur adapters are also available singly to convert the port of a butterfly for use with the evacuated tube system.

The butterfly system is for small veins that are difficult to draw with the evacuated tube system and standard evacuated tube system needle. The winged needle of the butterfly slides into a small surface vein. Instead of entering the vein at the usual 15-degree angle, the winged needle is inserted at approximately a 5-degree angle and then threaded into the vein. This procedure anchors the needle in the center of even a small vein. If the patient moves, the tubing gives flexibility so the needle will stay anchored and not pull out of the vein. The butterfly collection set works well on children and adults who have both small veins and the tendency to move while blood is being collected. The tubing also works as a pressure relief valve. An evacuated tube or syringe can be attached to the tubing and the vein will not collapse, as would normally occur. Drawing blood too quickly with a syringe will collapse the vein.

The butterfly system also provides the adaptability of initiating a draw with a syringe and then finishing it with the evacuated tube system. A syringe can be used for procedures that require a syringe sample, which is then removed and the evacuated tube system attached for multiple tube collection. Although the butterfly collection system has many benefits, it is not used for all collection. It is much more expensive than the needle system. The additional expense is unnecessary for the majority of venipunctures. Butterfly needles should be used only 10 to 15 percent of the time.

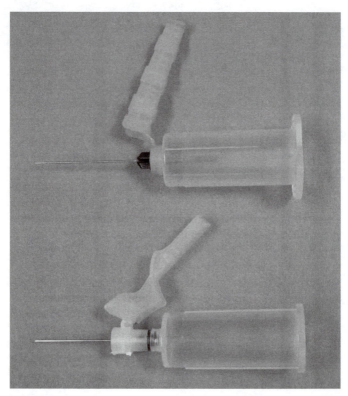

FIGURE 1.27 *Safety sleeve attached to holder (top). Safety sleeve attached to needle (bottom).*

Needle Safety

The Needlestick Safety and Prevention Act revised the Occupational Safety and Health Administration's (OSHA's) blood-borne pathogen standard. There are several parts to this law, but the part affecting the phlebotomist is the portion that addresses

FIGURE 1.28   *Butterfly needles for use with evacuated systems.*

"changes in technology that eliminate or reduce exposure to bloodborne pathogens." For the phlebotomist this means switching to what are known as "needlestick prevention devices." There are multiple devices on the market to be used with whatever type of needle is used. Figure 1.23 shows a safety sleeve that slides over the syringe needle. Figure 1.25 shows the safety sleeve attached to the needle and pushed by the thumb. Other devices attach to the holder instead of the needle. The locking cover protects the phlebotomist from needlesticks until the needle and holder can be discarded into a puncture-proof sharps container. Examples of butterfly safety devices are shown in Figure 1.28.

After use, the needle must remain attached to the holder and the entire needle and holder assembly must be discarded into a sharps container. The reasoning for not removing the needle is to avoid exposure of the part of the needle that punctures the tube. By not removing the needle from the holder, that end of the needle is shielded by the holder to prevent accidental needlestick.

Cleaning of the Draw Site

Antiseptics are used to clean the skin surface before a venipuncture, skin puncture, or arterial puncture. Antiseptics are chemical solutions that reduce the number of bacteria on the skin surface. Work practice controls dictate that to prevent infection of the patients or the health care worker, antiseptic solutions must be used. Types of antiseptics available include the following:

❖ 70 percent isopropyl alcohol either saturated into gauze or in prepackaged pads.

❖ Tincture of iodine or povidone-iodine. These come as pads or swabs and are mostly used for skin prep for blood cultures or arterial punctures.

❖ 2 percent chlorhexidine gluconate and 70 percent isopropyl alcohol, used for skin prep for blood cultures.

❖ Benzalkonium chloride, an alternate skin cleanser.

❖ Zephrin chloride, an alternate skin cleanser.

❖ Hydrogen peroxide, an alternate when there are allergies to alcohol.

Order of Drawing Tubes

With multiple draws using the evacuated system, the order of drawing the tubes is important. The recommended order of draw for direct collection into an evacuated system is as follows:

1. Blood culture bottle or yellow-stoppered blood culture tube (sterile procedure)

2. Coagulation tube (e.g., light blue stoppered)

3. Serum tube with or without clot activator or gel serum separator (e.g., red stoppered, red/black stoppered, plastic or glass)

4. Heparin tube with or without gel plasma separator (e.g., green stoppered)

5. EDTA tube (e.g., lavender stoppered)

6. Oxalate/fluoride, glycolytic inhibitor tube (e.g., gray stoppered)

If not all the tubes in the order of draw are to be collected, the order is started with the first tube needing collection. If all that needs to be collected is a green-stoppered tube and a lavender-stoppered tube, the green-stoppered tube is collected first, followed by the lavender-stoppered tube.

In orders for routine coagulation testing, such as PT and aPTT, which use a light blue–stoppered tube, the first tube collected can still be the light blue–stoppered tube.

There are two exceptions to this. When a butterfly is used, there is air in the tubing of the butterfly. For a light blue–stoppered tube that must be completely full, the air in the tubing will reduce the amount of blood in the tube. Therefore a plain-stoppered tube (no clot activator) or a light blue–stoppered tube must be drawn as a discard tube first to clear the air from the tubing. A second exception when a discard tube is collected first is with special coagulation testing. For special coagulation testing (factor assays), a plain red-stoppered tube (no clot activator) or a light blue–stoppered tube must be drawn as a discard tube first. This clears the draw site of a clotting substance called thromboplastin that is produced by the body as a result of the puncture.

The reasoning for an order of draw is that sterile collection tubes are collected first to prevent bacterial contamination. The anticoagulant tubes are drawn in the order indicated to avoid cross contamination of the anticoagulants. As a tube is pulled out of the evacuated tube holder, the needle is coated with a small amount of anticoagulant. This anticoagulant is then injected into the next tube drawn. If the heparin tube were drawn before the citrate tube, the citrate tube would have a small amount of heparin added to it and the patient's coagulation test results would appear as if the patient was on a blood thinner. An EDTA tube drawn before the green-stoppered tube can give a falsely elevated potassium.

Figure 1.29 shows the tubes in the correct order of draw.

FIGURE 1.29 *Tubes in the correct order of draw (blood culture, light blue, gel tube, green, lavender, gray).*

UNIT 2

Venipuncture Technique

Specimen Labeling

Proper patient identification and specimen labeling is as simple as drawing the correct patient's blood and labeling it with the correct name. All patient specimens must be positively identified on the primary container to avoid any errors in reporting of results, thereby affecting patient diagnosis or treatment. Improper patient identification and specimen labeling are the most common sources of error in phlebotomy. These errors can be easily avoided by following some simple steps.

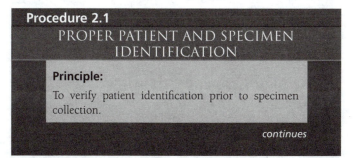

Procedure 2.1
PROPER PATIENT AND SPECIMEN IDENTIFICATION

Principle:
To verify patient identification prior to specimen collection.

continues

Procedure 2.1 *continued*

PROPER PATIENT AND SPECIMEN IDENTIFICATION

Procedure:

1. All requests for laboratory testing must have a requisition or computer labels. The requisition must include the patient's first and last name, test(s) requested, diagnosis, and name of ordering physician.

2. Every associate collecting a specimen from a patient checks two verifiers to ensure correct patient identification. Approach the patient in a professional and courteous manner. The patient will be unsure of what you are going to do. Explain the process you are going to perform and remember to focus on the patient and ignore outside distractions.

   A. Reading from the requisition or label, call the patient using the full name on the requisition or label.

   B. Before drawing the specimen, ask the patient to spell his or her last name and give the date of birth using the requisition as verification. A patient whose specimen is to be drawn for any blood bank procedure must be identified by an additional means besides the above procedure if he or she is an outpatient. The preferred identification sources for outpatients are as follows:

      a. A driver's license with a current address.

continues

Procedure 2.1 *continued*

PROPER PATIENT AND SPECIMEN IDENTIFICATION

   b. If the address is not current, then a driver's license and a personal check with the current address.

   c. Another form of identification with a current address.

C. If the patient is unable to verbally provide the information, a parent/guardian, nurse, or current picture ID may be used.

D. Computer-generated labels should be verified with the requisition for correct name before collecting the specimen.

3. After ensuring you have the correct patient, perform the venipuncture.

4. The specimen is labeled by the individual obtaining the specimen.

   A. The following must be included on the label:

   a. Patient's name (no nicknames).

   b. Medical record number, if available.

   c. Patient's birth date (for blood bank testing).

   d. Date and time collected.

   e. Source of the specimen (if other than blood).

   f. Initials of individuals obtaining the specimen.

continues

Procedure 2.1 *continued*

PROPER PATIENT AND SPECIMEN
IDENTIFICATION

    B. Aliquots or dilutions must be labeled with
    the following:

      a. Patient's name (no nicknames).

      b. Collection date.

      c. Type of specimen (plasma, serum, etc.).

    C. Timed collections must also be labeled with
    the time of collection and the type of col-
    lection (e.g., pre-, post-, fasting, one hour,
    two hour).

5. Read each label as it is attached to the tube
before leaving the patient. Compare one label
to another to ensure that all labels are for this
patient.

6. If computer labels are unavailable, labeling of
the tubes may be done by (a) addressograph
labels or (b) handwriting the patient's complete first and last name, hospital registration
number(s), room number, date and time of
draw as required by the test, and phlebotomist's initials.

7. If the patient does not have an identification
band on his or her wrist or ankle, or if the identification band is not correct, notify the nurse
or nursing unit secretary. Do not draw blood
unless the patient is wearing a correct identification band.

KEYS TO ACCURATE SPECIMEN LABELING

1. Specimen tubes should not be prelabeled.
2. Take laboratory labels to the bedside or outpatient location or hand write labels at the patient's side.
3. Compare each label to the others to verify that they are all for the same patient.
4. Compare the labels to the patient to verify that you are ready to draw a specimen from the correct patient.
5. Label all filled tubes BEFORE YOU LEAVE THE PATIENT. Tubes are to be labeled by the person doing the collecting.
6. Date and time each specimen collected.
7. Initial all tubes to verify all information on patient identification is correct.
8. Write the test name on the label.
9. Do not place unlabeled specimens in emesis basins, cups, or bags and label the container. If a specimen is held for possible testing later, it should be properly labeled and initialed by the associate who did the collection.
10. Labeled specimens are then bagged and sent to the proper laboratory.

Computer systems are replacing many of the manual requisitions. Hospitals now use computer systems consistently and only use manual systems when the computer system is down. Outpatient laboratory service centers also utilize computers to hold patient information for patients who return to the center and to print labels.

This helps the laboratory and the patient by having addresses and billing information readily available. Some laboratory computer systems are linked to the physician's office, so that the physician can order tests in the office and then have the patient go to the out-patient center to obtain the specimen. When the patient arrives, the laboratory is able to access the orders, collect the sample, and send the specimen to the testing laboratory. When the testing is completed, the physician can look up the patient's results wherever there is computer access.

Inaccuracy in patient identification and specimen labeling can cause serious problems for the patient.

> Specimens that are not correctly labeled can create problems:
> 1. The physician can miss a critical diagnosis.
> 2. An incorrect type of blood can be infused.
> 3. A patient can be incorrectly medicated due to invalid results.
> 4. Each mislabel opens the possibility of a lawsuit.
> 5. Injury or death to the patient can result.

Test Request Form

A test request form lists the information needed for the phlebotomist to complete the task. The patient's physician initiates the test request form. The following information should be included on the form:

❖ Patient's complete name and age or date of birth

❖ Patient identification number

❖ Date and time specimen is to be obtained

❖ Type of test to be collected

❖ Accessioning number

❖ Physician's name

- ❖ Department or location the work is to be done (on computer requests)

- ❖ Other information necessary to accurately collect the specimen, such as specific time of collection, fasting, etc.

- ❖ ICD-9 diagnosis codes for outpatients

Precautions in Blood Collection

The phlebotomist must be aware of various concerns that affect the phlebotomist or the outcome of the testing on a patient. Some of these are the result of procedural inconsistencies by the phlebotomist, whereas others are caused by the health of the patient. A few, as with latex allergies, can affect the health of the phlebotomist or the patient.

Hemoconcentration

Hemoconcentration is the increased concentration of constituents in the blood as a result of leaving the tourniquet on too long. The laboratory test results will then be invalid. This occurs because of a decrease in blood volume from fluid moving from the veins into the tissue. Those analytes that are too large to pass through the vascular wall are concentrated in the blood. Analytes such as calcium, cholesterol, lipids, drugs, steroids, and thyroid hormones increase.

To prevent hemoconcentration, do not leave the tourniquet on longer than one minute before venipuncture. If it takes longer than one minute to select a vein, remove the tourniquet for two minutes, then reapply the tourniquet.

Hematoma

A leakage of blood out of the vein during or after venipuncture causes a hematoma. A bruise will result. This accumulation of blood under the skin produces a discoloration on the skin, and the pressure of the buildup of blood can cause pain in the arm of the patient.

The following steps can help prevent a hematoma:

1. Remove the tourniquet before removing the needle.
2. Apply a small amount of pressure to the area after removal of the needle. Also tightly apply adhesive bandage over the gauze.
3. Do not use superficial veins.
4. Puncture only the uppermost wall of the vein. Do not puncture through both sides of the vein.
5. Make sure the needle fully punctures the uppermost wall of the vein. Partial penetration may allow the blood to leak into the tissue surrounding the vein.

Hemolysis

Hemolysis is the breaking or rupturing of the membrane of the red blood cells. The contents of the red blood cells then "contaminate" the serum or plasma to be tested. The serum or plasma appears slightly pink to a clear red in color. The laboratory tests are therefore inaccurate. Potassium is the first element to be affected.

The following steps can help prevent hemolysis:

1. Do not draw from a hematoma or bruised area.
2. Avoid using too small a needle, such as a 25 gauge.
3. Avoid drawing back the plunger of a syringe too forcefully.
4. Avoid foaming or frothing of the blood as it enters the syringe.
5. Let the alcohol on the puncture site air dry before inserting the needle.

Icteric Blood

Icteric blood, which results when a patient's serum or plasma contains a large amount of bilirubin because of jaundice, is blood that has a yellow to orange color. The patient's skin may also have the same yellow to orange color. This is caused by the patient's condition and not a blood collection error.

Lipemic Blood

Blood is lipemic when a large amount of fats and lipids are present in the blood, giving the serum and the plasma a white, milky color. This type of serum or plasma is known as lipemic. This is the result of the patient's condition and not a blood collection error.

Intravenous Line

Intravenous (IV) lines supply needed fluids and medicines to the patient. When an intravenous solution is being administered into one arm, blood should not be drawn from that arm. Blood drawn from the arm containing the intravenous solution has the potential to contaminate the blood specimen. Intravenous lines are inserted into a vein. The site can be anywhere from the back of the hand to farther up the arm. IV sites are generally not placed in the upper area of the arm but in any site below the upper arm. That makes the upper arm area very tempting to draw blood from because the veins can be felt in the upper arm and the IV is in the lower part of the arm. Venous blood is flowing up the arm from the hand to the shoulder. The IV solution is flowing in that direction. Any blood drawn in a site above the IV will contain the IV solution. The IV solution will be in a high concentration because it has not had a chance to circulate through the body. As a result, the laboratory test results will be higher or lower depending on the contents of the IV solution.

To avoid this kind of error, the phlebotomist should look for a blood-drawing site in the opposite arm. Occasionally, an IV is running in both arms and no site can be found except in the area of the IV. Satisfactory samples can be drawn below the IV by following several precautions. Preferably have the IV shut off for at least

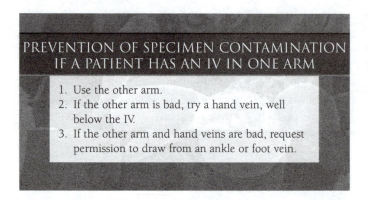

PREVENTION OF SPECIMEN CONTAMINATION
IF A PATIENT HAS AN IV IN ONE ARM

1. Use the other arm.
2. If the other arm is bad, try a hand vein, well below the IV.
3. If the other arm and hand veins are bad, request permission to draw from an ankle or foot vein.

two minutes before venipuncture. (The phlebotomist must never shut off a running IV. The nurse or physician of that patient must make the decision to shut off an IV, even temporarily.) Apply the tourniquet below the IV site. Select a vein other than the one with the IV. Perform the venipuncture. Draw 7 to 10 milliliters of blood and discard this blood to clear any IV solutions from the arm before test samples are collected.

Vascular Access Device (Line)

A vascular access device (VAD), also called an indwelling line or heparin/saline well, consists of tubing inserted into a main vein or artery (Figure 2.1). It is used primarily for administering fluids and medications, monitoring pressures, and drawing blood. Specially trained individuals should be the only persons with VAD access. Because lines are routinely flushed with heparin or saline, a discard volume of blood must be drawn. For adults, a discard volume of 7 to 10 milliliters is drawn. If the proper discard volume is not drawn, the laboratory test results will be erroneous.

This procedure is generally reserved for the nurse or physician of the patient and cannot be completed by the phlebotomist.

FIGURE 2.1 *Heparin/saline well.*

Handwashing

Handwashing is the single most important means of preventing the spread of infection. Hands must be washed under running water with soap and vigorous rubbing. When the soap is rinsed off, the water should flow from the wrists to the fingertips. Waterless disinfectant cleaners are used only when running water is not available. See Procedure 1.1 for proper handwashing technique.

Latex Allergy

Latex, which is made from the natural rubber of trees, can be found in many household and health care products. Balloons, toys, garden hoses, rubber gloves, tourniquets, intravenous tubing, blood pressure cuffs, and bandages are a few of the products that can contain latex. Allergies to latex have been on the increase as there is more exposure to latex products. Phlebotomists are at high risk due to their constant exposure to latex tourniquets and latex gloves.

Reactions to latex can vary with the individual, from itchy irritation to redness and swelling, progressing to thickened skin, pimples, or skin blisters that ooze. This is the typical, less serious type IV allergy to latex due to contact dermatitis. Symptoms begin 24 to 72 hours after exposure and can continue for several days. With each additional exposure, the symptoms become more advanced.

Type I latex allergy is more serious. This is an immunological reaction that is caused by the penetration of the natural latex proteins into the skin. These proteins cause a production of antibodies to latex and increases with each subsequent exposure. As the allergy becomes more severe, the symptoms may include nausea, low blood pressure, and respiratory distress. If the latex allergen is introduced directly into the blood, anaphylactic shock is possible. This can be life threatening.

To prevent allergic reactions, exposure to latex must be eliminated. There is no cure for latex allergy, only prevention of exposure. This prevention of exposure is not only for the phlebotomist but also for the patient. If the phlebotomist has a latex allergy, latex gloves or tourniquets must not be used. If the patient has a latex allergy, the phlebotomist must avoid any type of latex contact to the patient. This includes the tourniquet, latex gloves, blood pressure cuffs, and adhesive bandages.

Latex allergies do not always come in the form of direct contact to the skin. The powder in the gloves disperses the latex into the air, and then the phlebotomist or the patient inhales the powder, producing a respiratory reaction. A less serious form of powder allergy occurs when powder gets in the eyes and the eyes become irritated and swollen. Most health care providers are switching to powder-free gloves to avoid problems.

Collecting the Venipuncture Blood Sample

Positioning the Patient

The position of the patient is critical for proper patient blood collection. The best position is the position that is comfortable for the patient and the phlebotomist. Proper positioning of the patient makes the patient feel more at ease, and the phlebotomist is better able to perform the venipuncture. In most critical care situations the patient is reclining, the ideal position to draw blood. If the patient is ambulatory, then proper patient position must be maintained.

Before a patient's blood is drawn, ask the patient if he or she has ever had any problems with blood being taken. Usually one of two situations must be addressed:

1. The patient does not have a problem with having blood drawn:
   a. The patient must be in a seated or reclining position before any attempt is made to draw blood.
   b. Do not allow the patient to sit on a tall stool or stand while drawing blood. There is always the possibility that the patient will faint (syncope) and injure himself or herself.
   c. The sitting position requires a chair with adequate arm supports that are adjustable for the best venipuncture position.
   d. A pillow may be required to help support the patient's arm by keeping it straight for easier venous access.
2. The patient might faint (syncope):
   a. Have the patient lie down whenever he or she indicates apprehension or if the patient has fainted while having blood drawn before.
   b. The reclining position is the ideal position from which to draw a blood sample from the patient.

Selecting the Appropriate Venipuncture Site

The appropriate venipuncture site can vary depending on the patient. The usual site that is first checked is the upper (antecubital fossa) region of the arm. The primary vein used in the upper arm is the median cubital vein. This is usually the prominent vein in the middle of the bend of the arm (Figure 2.2).

Basilic

Cephalic

Median Cubital

Median

FIGURE 2.2 *Superficial veins in the arm.*

The basilic, cephalic, or median veins can be used as an alternative. If these veins are not accessible or not prominent enough to obtain a blood sample from, go to the back of the hand to determine other possibilities. The veins in the back of the hand have the tendency to "roll" more than the arm veins because they are not supported by as much tissue and are closer to the surface. To avoid this, the vein must be held in place by the index finger and the thumb while a smaller gauge needle or a butterfly is used. The hand veins are best accessed with a 3- to 5-milliliter syringe with a 22-gauge needle or a 23-gauge butterfly. The wrist veins are also an alternative but generally are much more painful than the other sites. The wrist vein that is accessible is the vein that is in line with the thumb. By following the thumb up to the wrist area, a predominant vein on top of the wrist is usually found. The foot and ankle veins may also be used if the patient's physician gives permission. The veins in the foot or ankle also have the tendency to roll.

If all the alternatives have failed to reveal an acceptable venipuncture site, then a more experienced phlebotomist should check. If venous access is not possible, determine if it is possible to collect the sample from a fingerstick.

ORDER FOR CHECKING FOR BEST AVAILABLE VENIPUNCTURE SITE

1. Upper arm
2. Hand
3. Wrist (vein in line with the thumb)
4. Ankle or foot

Vein Stimulation

The tourniquet makes the veins more prominent by restricting the venous flow and inhibiting the arterial flow of blood in the arm. The tourniquet is a soft, pliable, rubber strip approximately 1 inch wide by 15 to 18 inches long. The tourniquet can be either latex or non-latex for patients or phlebotomists with latex allergies (Figure 2.3).

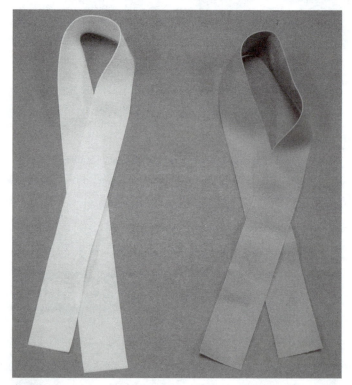

FIGURE 2.3 *Latex tourniquet (left), nonlatex tourniquet (right).*

The strip tourniquet is best for all conditions. The rubber strip can easily be released with one hand. Because it is about 1 inch wide, it does not cut into the patient's arm but distributes the pressure. Tourniquets are inexpensive enough that they can be discarded after each use. When tying a tourniquet, the ends should be pointed upward to prevent the ends from falling down on the venipuncture site.

Procedure 2.2 outlines the procedure for tying and releasing a tourniquet.

Procedure 2.2

TYING AND RELEASING A TOURNIQUET

Principle:

To properly tie a tourniquet to constrict blood flow for venous access but not compromise circulation.

Procedure:

1. Determine if you can use a latex tourniquet or will need a nonlatex tourniquet.

2. Inspect the patient's arms for the most likely vein to use.

3. Wrap the tourniquet around the arm 3 to 4 inches above the likely venipuncture site. Keep the tourniquet flat to minimize the discomfort to the patient (Figure 2.4).

continues

Procedure 2.2 *continued*

TYING AND RELEASING A TOURNIQUET

4. Stretch the tourniquet, bring both ends to the front of the patient, and cross the ends of the tourniquet (Figure 2.5).

5. While holding the ends tight, tuck one portion of the tourniquet under the other. This is usually the end of the tourniquet that is the lower of the two (nearest the hand) (Figure 2.6).

6. By tucking the lower of the two ends, the loose ends of the tourniquet are facing upward and should not be a hindrance to the venipuncture (Figure 2.7).

7. The tourniquet should now cause the veins to be more prominent.

8. To release the tourniquet, pull on the end of the tourniquet that you tucked.

FIGURE 2.4 *Wrap the tourniquet around the arm 3 to 4 inches above the likely venipuncture site. Keep the tourniquet flat to minimize the discomfort to the patient.*

FIGURE 2.5 *Stretch the tourniquet and bring both ends to the front of the patient and cross the ends of the tourniquet.*

continues

Procedure 2.2   *continued*

TYING AND RELEASING A TOURNIQUET

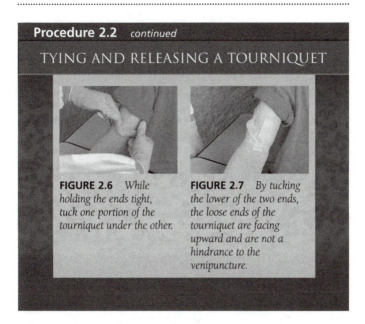

FIGURE 2.6 *While holding the ends tight, tuck one portion of the tourniquet under the other.*

FIGURE 2.7 *By tucking the lower of the two ends, the loose ends of the tourniquet are facing upward and are not a hindrance to the venipuncture.*

A tourniquet must be used to assist the phlebotomist in feeling a vein. The tourniquet is applied 3 to 4 inches above the puncture site. It is applied tightly enough to stop the flow of blood in the veins but not so tightly as to prevent the flow of blood in the arteries. This is similar to damming a small stream. When the stream is dammed, the water forms a pond in front of the dam. With the tourniquet applied, the veins fill with blood, pooling in the veins below the tourniquet. This pooling of blood makes the veins more prominent. The vein must be palpated with the tip of the index finger to determine its depth and size. Feel for and trace the path of the vein several times. Avoid using the thumb because it has a pulse and is not as sensitive as the rest of the fingers. The vein feels soft and bouncy to the touch. The roundness of the vein and the direction it follows may be determined. All veins are not straight up and down the arm. If no veins become prominent, retie the tourniquet tighter but not so tightly as to stop the flow of arterial blood into the arm. If the tourniquet is tied tightly enough to stop arterial blood flow, the patient will no longer have a pulse in the wrist. If this occurs, immediately remove the tourniquet, because this indicates that blood has ceased below the tourniquet. If a vein cannot be felt, several methods may be used to stimulate vein prominence.

The tourniquet often causes greater discomfort for patients than the venipuncture itself. Ideally the tourniquet should be removed as soon as blood flow is established. The act of removing the tourniquet may move the needle or vein just enough so that no more blood can be obtained and a second venipuncture must be performed. It is recommended to wait until just before the needle is removed from the patient to remove the tourniquet. If the tourniquet is not removed before the needle is removed, the patient will bleed heavily. Blood will be forced out of the needle hole and into the surrounding tissue, resulting in a hematoma.

METHODS OF VEIN STIMULATION

1. Position the arm lower than the patient.
2. Reapply the tourniquet.
3. Massage the arm in an upward motion.
4. Use a blood pressure cuff in place of the tourniquet.
5. Warm the venipuncture site with a warming device or a warm washcloth.

There are several situations in which venipuncture should be avoided (Figure 2.8). If the "vein" that is felt has a pulsing action to it, this indicates that it is an artery, not a vein, and the vessel should not be punctured. Tendons can be deceptive and give the appearance of a vein. They do not have the soft, bouncy feel and are hard to the touch. Puncturing a tendon gives no blood return and is painful to the patient. There are also nerves that run the length of the arm. The nerves cannot be seen or felt,

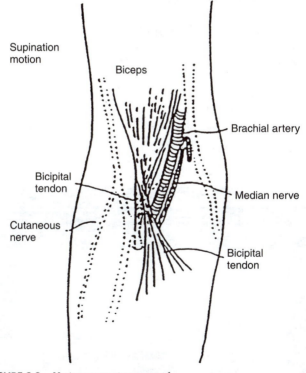

FIGURE 2.8 *Venipuncture sites to avoid.*

but by avoiding deep, probing venipunctures, the chance of touching a nerve is diminished. If the patient complains that the venipuncture is extremely painful, it is best to stop and try another site.

In edematous arms that are swollen due to fluid in the tissue, veins will not be prominent and the tourniquet will not be effective because of the swelling. Using the tourniquet in this instance creates the potential for tissue damage. It leaves a temporary indentation in the arm. Areas of scarring should also be avoided due to possible injury or excessive pain to the patient. Specimens collected from an area of a hematoma may produce erroneous test results. If another vein site is not available, the specimen is collected distal from the hematoma. Arms with fistulas should also be avoided. Because of the potential for harm to the patient due to lymphostasis, the arm on the side of a mastectomy should be avoided. If the patient has had a double mastectomy, a physician should be consulted prior to drawing the blood. Generally the phlebotomist draws from the side of the oldest mastectomy.

VENIPUNCTURE SITES TO AVOID

1. Above an IV site
2. Pulsating arterial areas
3. Tendons or veins without a soft bounce
4. Nerves
5. Edematous areas
6. Side of a mastectomy

Syringe Specimen Collection

The patient has been identified, paperwork and tubes verified, and equipment assembled, and the patient is in a comfortable position. The next step is to tie the tourniquet. Have the patient close the hand, and then select a vein. If possible, place the patient's arm in a downward position. After locating an acceptable vein, mentally map the location. Set mental sights on the vein by visualizing the puncture site as the target. It might be slightly over from this freckle and a little down from that wrinkle. Set those mental sights for an accurate puncture. Cleanse the site with a gauze pad wet with 70 percent isopropyl alcohol solution. A commercially pre-pared alcohol pad or one with 0.5 percent chlorhexidine in alco-hol may also be used. The skin is cleansed in a circular motion from the center to the outside. The area is allowed to air dry to pre-vent hemolysis of the specimen and to prevent the patient from feeling a burning sensation during blood collection.

Some authorities suggest donning gloves first and then palpating for the vein. This technique is required for the patient who is isolated due to a communicable disease and is good practice for all patients. Standard precautions require that personal protective equipment be worn when there is a chance of coming in contact with blood and body fluid. If the patient has veins that are difficult to palpate, gloves may be donned after the site has been palpated and before the cleansing. To avoid forgetting the best location of the collection site, palpate the vein 1 to 2 inches above and below the intended punc-ture site. It helps the phlebotomist feel that the vein is located in a straight line, and these points can be used to "reset" the mental crosshairs without contaminating the venipuncture site. Goggles and a mask must be worn if there is a potential for blood spatter.

The syringe technique is used less often than the evacuated system. The techniques developed in the syringe method are building blocks for the evacuated tube technique and all other techniques that the phlebotomist uses for obtaining a blood sample.

CORRECT HAND POSITION TO HOLD A SYRINGE

1. The needle is attached to the syringe.
2. The syringe and needle system is held in the dominant hand and cradled on the four fingers.
3. The thumb is then placed on top of the syringe.
4. A right-handed person holds the syringe in the right hand, leaving the left hand to pull on the plunger. A left-handed person does the opposite.
5. With the syringe held in this position, turn it slightly so the bevel of the needle is facing up (Figure 2.9).
6. Hold the hand in such a position that by tilting the point of the needle down slightly, the needle enters the skin at a 15-degree angle and about ¼ inch below the point the phlebotomist felt the vein (Figure 2.10).

FIGURE 2.9   *Correct hand position to hold a syringe.*

A. Location vein is felt
B. Point needle enters skin
A - B. Approximately one-fourth inch. The deeper the vein the greater the distance.

FIGURE 2.10 *Position at which to enter the skin. Left, Location at which the vein is felt (A); point at which needle enters skin (B). Right, Distance between A and B is approximately ¼ inch. The deeper the vein, the greater the distance.*

The syringe is ideal for small blood samples in fragile surface veins such as veins in the back of the hand. Procedure 2.3 explains venipuncture with a syringe.

When a syringe is used, the blood obtained must be placed in appropriate containers. Aliquot the blood into evacuated tubes according to step 25 of Procedure 2.3. Do not remove the rubber stoppers. Running blood down the side of the tube after removing the stopper is not recommended because aerosols and splattering of blood can occur. Do not hold the tube in your hand as you puncture the stopper. There is the potential for missing the stopper or slipping off the stopper and puncturing yourself. The best method is to place the tubes in a test tube rack or use a transfer device.

Procedure 2.3

VENIPUNCTURE BY SYRINGE

Principle:

To obtain venous blood acceptable for laboratory testing as required by a physician. Venous blood collected is to be aliquoted into evacuated tubes and/or special collection containers.

Materials:

Disposable gloves.

Goggles and mask.

Syringe, varies in size.

Disposable needle for syringe, 21 or 22 gauge.

Evacuated tube(s) or special collection tube(s).

Tourniquet.

70 percent isopropyl alcohol swab.

Gauze or cotton balls.

Adhesive bandage or tape.

Sharps container.

Transfer device.

Procedure:

1. Identify the patient. Inpatient: Verify identification bracelet name and hospital number with computer requisition information. Outpatient: Ask the patient's name and verify with computer label or identification numbers.

continues

Procedure 2.3 *continued*

VENIPUNCTURE BY SYRINGE

2. If a fasting specimen is required, ask the patient when he or she last ate. Explain the procedure to the patient.

3. Wash hands.

4. Don gloves. Putting on gloves may be delayed until step 12 for a nonisolation patient.

5. Open the sterile needle and syringe packages, attaching the needle if necessary.

6. Prevent the plunger from sticking by pulling it halfway out and pushing it all the way in one time (breathe the syringe).

7. Select the proper tube(s) to transfer the blood to after collection.

8. Apply the tourniquet.

9. Ask the patient to close the hand. The patient must not be allowed to pump the hand. Pumping of the hand changes the values of the laboratory tests being collected due to hemoconcentration. Place the patient's arm in a downward position if possible.

10. Select a vein, noting the location and direction of the vein (Figure 2.11).

11. Clean the venipuncture site with a 70 percent isopropyl alcohol swab in a circular motion from the center outward (Figure 2.12).

12. Don gloves if not done in step 4.

continues

Procedure 2.3 *continued*

VENIPUNCTURE BY SYRINGE

13. Do not touch the venipuncture site. If there is a potential for blood spatter, goggles and a mask must be worn.

14. Draw the skin taut with your thumb. Place the thumb 1 to 2 inches below the puncture site (Figure 2.13).

15. With the bevel up, line up the needle with the vein and perform the venipuncture (Figure 2.14).

FIGURE 2.11 *Feel for a vein.*

FIGURE 2.12 *Clean site with isopropyl alcohol.*

FIGURE 2.13 *Draw skin taut with your thumb.*

FIGURE 2.14 *Perform venipuncture. Secure the syringe with one hand and pull on the syringe plunger with the other hand.*

continues

Procedure 2.3 *continued*

VENIPUNCTURE BY SYRINGE

16. Do not enter the vein at the exact location at which the vein is felt. Enter the vein approximately $\frac{1}{4}$ inch below the vein location. The location where the vein was palpated is the point where the bevel of the needle must be in the vein (see Figure 2.10). Push the needle into the skin. A sensation of resistance will be followed by easy penetration as the vein is entered. This is known as feeling the "pop." Once this point is reached, stop and do not move.

17. Using the opposite hand, pull on the plunger of the syringe. Pull gently and only as fast as the syringe will fill with blood. Pulling too hard or fast will cause temporary collapse of the vein. If the vein does collapse, stop pulling on the plunger and let the vein refill with blood.

18. Pull the plunger back until the desired amount of blood has been obtained.

19. Ask the patient to open the hand.

20. Release the tourniquet.

21. Lightly place a gauze square or cotton ball above the venipuncture site.

22. Remove the needle from the arm.

23. Activate the safety shield over the needle.

24. Apply pressure to the site for three to five minutes. The patient may assist if able by elevating the arm above the heart level. The patient should not bend his or her arm.

continues

Procedure 2.3 *continued*

VENIPUNCTURE BY SYRINGE

25. Aliquot the blood into the appropriate tube(s). Always follow the order of draw when filling tubes. Attach a transfer device to the syringe, and fill evacuated tubes through the transfer device (Figure 2.15). Alternately, place the appropriate tube(s) in a test tube rack. Puncture the stopper of the evacuated tube with the syringe needle and allow blood to enter the tube until flow stops (Figure 2.16). Invert the tube(s) if any anticoagulant is present.

26. Immediately discard intact syringe and needle in a sharps container.

27. Discard gauze and other waste in biohazard containers.

28. Label all tubes before leaving the patient's room.

29. Apply an adhesive bandage.

FIGURE 2.15 *Use a transfer device to fill evacuated tubes.*

continues

Procedure 2.3 *continued*

VENIPUNCTURE BY SYRINGE

FIGURE 2.16 *Puncture the stopper of evacuated tube with syringe needle and allow blood to enter tube until flow stops.*

The tube will fill itself; do not force the blood into the tube. This technique maintains the proper ratio of blood to anticoagulant. Immediately upon filling, mix any anticoagulant tubes.

Evacuated Tube Specimen Collection

The evacuated tube system is an improvement over the syringe method, yet maintains many similarities. When using the syringe method, as the syringe plunger is pulled, a vacuum is created. With the evacuated tube system, the vacuum is already in the tube. Another advantage of the evacuated tube system is that with multiple blood samples, syringes do not need to be changed; only the tubes need to be changed. This creates the advantage of a closed system; there is no transferring of blood from the syringe to a tube.

The similarity between the evacuated tube system and the syringe system is that the holder and needle are held in the same manner. A syringe is held in a manner to allow the phlebotomist access to pull on the plunger. In the evacuated system, access must be allowed for one tube to be pulled out and another inserted. The hand that pulled on the plunger of the syringe is the hand that changes tubes with the evacuated system.

The procedure for venipuncture with the evacuated tube system follows the same steps as the syringe method, with only slight variation (Procedure 2.4).

Butterfly Collection System

The butterfly system maintains many similarities to the evacuated system. The butterfly provides the convenience of evacuated tubes but offers the flexibility to use a syringe if needed. What most phlebotomists like about the butterfly system is that when the needle enters the vein there is a "flash" of blood where the tubing is attached to the needle. This flash gives the phlebotomist a visual that the vein has been accessed. For an experienced phlebotomist, this visual flash is not necessary for most patients and a regular needle can be used.

Procedure 2.4

VENIPUNCTURE BY EVACUATED TUBE SYSTEM

Principle:

To obtain venous blood acceptable for laboratory testing as required by a physician. Venous blood is collected by evacuated tubes. The volume of blood is dependent on size of the tube and on test requirements.

Materials:

Gloves.

Goggles and mask.

Evacuated tube holder.

Disposable needle for evacuated system, 20, 21, or 22 gauge.

Evacuated tube(s) or special collection tube(s).

Tourniquet.

70 percent isopropyl alcohol swab.

Gauze or cotton balls.

Adhesive bandage or tape.

Sharps container.

Procedure:

1. Identify the patient. Inpatient: Verify identification bracelet name and hospital number with computer requisition information. Outpatient: Ask patient's name and verify with computer label or identification numbers.

continues

Procedure 2.4 *continued*

VENIPUNCTURE BY EVACUATED TUBE SYSTEM

2. If a fasting specimen is required, ask the patient when he or she last ate.

3. Wash hands.

4. Don gloves. Putting on gloves may be delayed until step 12 for nonisolation patients.

5. Collect equipment.

6. Break the needle seal. Thread the appropriate needle into the holder using the needle sheath as a wrench.

7. Insert the tube into the holder until the needle slightly enters the stopper. Avoid pushing the needle beyond the recessed guideline, because a loss of vacuum may result. If the tube retracts slightly, leave it in the retracted position to avoid prematurely puncturing the rubber stopper.

8. Apply the tourniquet.

9. Ask the patient to close the hand. The patient must not be allowed to pump the hand. Pumping of the hand changes the values of the laboratory tests being collected due to hemoconcentration. If possible, place the patient's arm in a downward position.

10. Feel for a vein, noting the location and direction of the vein (Figure 2.17).

11. Clean the venipuncture site with a 70 percent isopropyl alcohol swab in a circular motion from the center outward.

continues

Procedure 2.4 *continued*

VENIPUNCTURE BY EVACUATED TUBE SYSTEM

12. Don gloves if not done in step 4.

13. Do not touch the venipuncture site. If there is a potential for blood spatter, goggles and a mask must be worn.

14. Draw the skin taut with your thumb and index finger. Place the index finger at the point the vein was felt and the thumb 1 to 2 inches below the puncture site.

15. With the bevel up, line up the needle with the vein while holding the skin taut. Perform the venipuncture (Figure 2.18). Remove your hand from drawing the skin taut (Figure 2.19). Grasp the flange of the evacuated tube holder, and push the tube forward until the butt end of the needle punctures the stopper (Figure 2.20). You should not change hands while performing the venipuncture. The hand you perform the venipuncture with is the hand that holds the evacuated tube holder. This provides stability

FIGURE 2.17 *Feel for vein direction and location.*

FIGURE 2.18 *Insert needle while holding skin taut.*

continues

Procedure 2.4 *continued*

VENIPUNCTURE BY EVACUATED TUBE SYSTEM

FIGURE 2.19 *Remove hand from holding skin taut.*

FIGURE 2.20 *Insert tubes into holder in the correct order of draw.*

for the phlebotomist and the comfort of human touch to the patient. The opposite hand manipulates the tubes.

16. Do not enter the vein at the exact location at which the vein is felt. Enter the vein approximately ¼ inch below the vein location. The location that the vein was palpated is the point where the bevel of the needle must be in the vein. Push the needle into the skin. A sensation of resistance will be followed by easy penetration as the vein is entered. This is known as feeling the "pop." Once this point is reached, stop and do not move.

17. Fill the tube until the vacuum is exhausted and blood flow into the tube ceases (Figure 2.21). This ensures the proper blood-to-anticoagulant ratio. Remove the tube from the holder. While securely grasping the evacuated tube holder with one hand, use the other hand to change

continues

Procedure 2.4   *continued*

VENIPUNCTURE BY EVACUATED TUBE SYSTEM

FIGURE 2.21   *Fill tube until vacuum is exhausted.*

the tubes. The shutoff valve re-covers the point, stopping the flow of blood until the next tube of blood is inserted. Fill the remaining tubes following the correct order of draw.

18. Immediately after filling, invert each tube that contains an additive. Gently inverting the tube 5 to 10 times provides adequate mixing without causing hemolysis. Do not shake the tube.

19. Ask the patient to open the hand.

20. Release the tourniquet.

21. Lightly place a gauze square or cotton ball above venipuncture site.

22. Remove the needle from the arm. Be certain that the last tube drawn has been removed from the holder before removing the needle. This prevents blood droplets from falling off the tip of the needle.

23. Activate the safety shield on the needle.

continues

Procedure 2.4 *continued*

VENIPUNCTURE BY EVACUATED TUBE SYSTEM

24. Dispose of the needle and holder in a sharps container.

25. Apply pressure to the site for three to five minutes. The patient may assist if able and elevate the arm above the heart to reduce blood flow.

26. Label all tubes at the patient's side before leaving the patient's room.

27. Apply an adhesive bandage.

Using the butterfly system with each patient is more costly than the regular needle system. Therefore the butterfly system should be limited to patients who have small veins.

One concern with the butterfly collection system is the air in the tubing after the venipuncture has been performed. The first tube pulls the air from the tubing, resulting in a tube that is approximately 0.5 milliliter short of the correct amount of blood. This is not a problem for most tests. However, a light blue–stoppered tube must maintain the 1:9 ratio of anticoagulant to blood for accurate testing from that tube. When the first tube to be collected is a light blue–stoppered tube, a discard tube (a red-stoppered tube with no additive or another light blue–stoppered tube) must be collected to pull the air from the tubing. A discard tube that has any additive cannot be used because of the carryover of the additive into the light blue–stoppered tube.

The procedure for venipuncture with the butterfly system follows the same steps as for the evacuated tube system, with only slight variation.

Procedure 2.5

VENIPUNCTURE BY BUTTERFLY NEEDLE SYSTEM

Principle:

To obtain venous blood acceptable for laboratory testing as required by a physician. The amount of the venous blood specimen is dependent on the size of the tube and the test requirements.

Materials:

Gloves.

Goggles and mask.

Evacuated tube holder.

Butterfly needle system, 21- or 23-gauge needle with or without Leur adapter.

Syringe if not using Leur adapter on butterfly needle.

Evacuated tube(s) or special collection tube(s).

Tourniquet.

70 percent isopropyl alcohol swab.

Gauze or cotton balls.

Adhesive bandage or tape.

Sharps container.

Procedure:

1. Identify the patient. Inpatient: Verify identification bracelet name and hospital number with computer requisition information. Outpatient: Ask the patient's name and verify with computer label or identification numbers.

continues

Procedure 2.5 *continued*

VENIPUNCTURE BY BUTTERFLY NEEDLE SYSTEM

2. If a fasting specimen is required, ask the patient when he or she last ate.

3. Wash hands.

4. Don gloves. Putting on gloves may be delayed until step 12 for nonisolation patients.

5. Collect equipment.

6. Open the package of the butterfly needle system with evacuated tube Leur adapter. Thread the Leur needle into the holder.

7. Insert the tube into the holder until the needle slightly enters the stopper. Avoid pushing the needle beyond the recessed guideline, because a loss of vacuum may result. If the tube retracts slightly, leave it in the retracted position.

8. Apply the tourniquet.

9. Ask the patient to close the hand. The patient must not be allowed to pump the hand. Pumping of the hand changes the values of the laboratory tests being collected due to hemoconcentration. If possible, place the patient's arm in a downward position.

10. Feel for a vein, noting the location and direction of the vein (Figure 2.22).

11. Clean the venipuncture site with a 70 percent isopropyl alcohol swab in a circular motion from the center outward (Figure 2.23).

12. Don gloves if not done in step 4.

continues

Procedure 2.5 *continued*

VENIPUNCTURE BY BUTTERFLY NEEDLE SYSTEM

FIGURE 2.22 *Feel for a vein.*

FIGURE 2.23 *Clean the venipuncture site with isopropyl alcohol.*

13. Do not touch the venipuncture site. If there is a potential for blood spatter, goggles and a mask must be worn.

14. Draw the skin taut with your thumb and index finger. Place the index finger at the point the vein was felt and the thumb 1 to 2 inches below the puncture site.

15. Hold the butterfly with the bevel up. Line up the needle with the vein and perform the venipuncture (Figure 2.24).

16. Do not enter the vein at the exact location at which the vein is felt. Enter the vein approximately ¼ inch below the vein location. The location where the vein was palpated is the point where the bevel of the needle must be in the vein. Push the needle into the skin. A sensation of resistance will be followed by easy penetration as the vein is entered. This is known as feeling the "pop." Once this point is reached, you

continues

Procedure 2.5 *continued*

VENIPUNCTURE BY BUTTERFLY NEEDLE SYSTEM

should see a flash of blood in the needle tubing (Figure 2.25). Stop and do not move.

17. Remove your hand from drawing the skin taut. Grasp the flange of the evacuated tube holder and push the tube forward until the butt end of the needle punctures the stopper (Figure 2.26). Do not change hands while performing the venipuncture. The hand performing the venipuncture is the hand that holds the butterfly needle. The opposite hand manipulates the tubes.

18. Fill the tube until the vacuum is exhausted and blood flow into the tube ceases. This ensures the proper blood-to-anticoagulant ratio. Due to air in the tubing, a loss of approximately 0.5 milliliter will result when collecting the initial evacuated tube.

19. When the blood flow ceases, remove the tube from the holder. Insert the next tube into the

FIGURE 2.24 *Perform venipuncture.*

FIGURE 2.25 *When needle enters the vein, you should see a "flash" of blood.*

continues

Procedure 2.5 *continued*

VENIPUNCTURE BY BUTTERFLY NEEDLE SYSTEM

holder according to the correct order of draw. The shutoff valve re-covers the point, stopping the flow of blood until the next tube of blood is inserted.

20. Immediately after drawing, invert each tube that contains an additive. Gently inverting the tube 5 to 10 times provides adequate mixing without causing hemolysis. Do not shake the tubes.

21. Ask the patient to open the hand.

22. Release the tourniquet (Figure 2.27).

23. Remove the last tube to draw from the holder (Figure 2.28).

24. Lightly place a gauze square or cotton ball above the venipuncture site.

25. Remove the needle from the arm. Be certain that the last tube drawn has been removed from the holder before removing needle (Figure 2.29). This prevents blood from dripping out of the tip of the needle.

FIGURE 2.26 *Insert evacuated tube into holder.*

FIGURE 2.27 *Release tourniquet.*

continues

Procedure 2.5 *continued*

VENIPUNCTURE BY BUTTERFLY NEEDLE SYSTEM

FIGURE 2.28 *Remove the last tube from holder.*

FIGURE 2.29 *Remove butterfly needle from the arm.*

FIGURE 2.30 *Activate safety shield.*

26. Activate the safety shield on the needle (Figure 2.30).

27. Apply pressure to the site for three to five minutes. The patient may assist if able. The arm should be elevated to reduce blood flow.

28. Dispose of the needle and holder in a sharps container. When disposing, insert the needle end of the device first and allow the tubing and holder to drop into the container.

continues

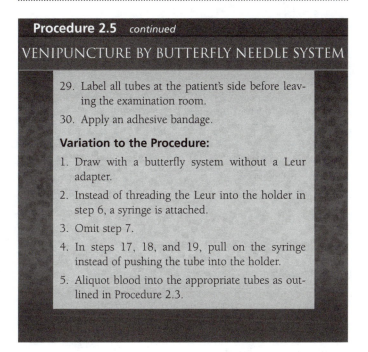

Procedure 2.5 *continued*

VENIPUNCTURE BY BUTTERFLY NEEDLE SYSTEM

29. Label all tubes at the patient's side before leaving the examination room.

30. Apply an adhesive bandage.

Variation to the Procedure:

1. Draw with a butterfly system without a Leur adapter.

2. Instead of threading the Leur into the holder in step 6, a syringe is attached.

3. Omit step 7.

4. In steps 17, 18, and 19, pull on the syringe instead of pushing the tube into the holder.

5. Aliquot blood into the appropriate tubes as outlined in Procedure 2.3.

The Unsuccessful Venipuncture

When a blood sample cannot be obtained, it may be necessary to change the position of the needle. Rotate the needle half a turn. The bevel of the needle may be against the wall of the vein. If the needle has not penetrated the vein far enough, advance it farther into the vein. Only advance slightly; a small change may be the difference between a failed and a successful venipuncture. If the needle has penetrated too far into the vein, pull back a little. Always "bail out" slowly when the venipuncture has been unsuccessful. The blood often may start coming just as it seems the needle is ready to come out of the skin. The tube used may not have sufficient vacuum. Try another tube before withdrawing needle.

Probing of the site is not recommended. Probing is painful to the patient and may cause a hematoma. Never attempt a venipuncture more than two times. If a blood sample cannot be obtained after two attempts, perform a microcollection if possible. Otherwise have another person attempt the draw. Notify the patient's physician if two attempts have been unsuccessful and a microcollection is not possible.

Criteria for Re-collection or Rejection of a Specimen

The primary goal of the phlebotomist collecting the blood sample is to provide an acceptable specimen for laboratory testing as required by the physician. There are certain general criteria that must be met for a specimen to be acceptable. If the criteria are not met, the specimen is rejected and another venipuncture of the patient must be performed.

This list is not inclusive. The type of specimen that is acceptable and the volume required is determined by the procedure ordered. Another specimen is often done to recheck results on a patient. The quality control checks done by the laboratory may indicate that the results are valid. If the results do not agree with what the physician feels is the patient's diagnosis, the blood specimen may need to be redrawn to confirm the results. This is accomplished by either retesting the specimen or collecting another sample. This will either reconfirm that the correct specimen was drawn or indicate that the patient's test results changed significantly.

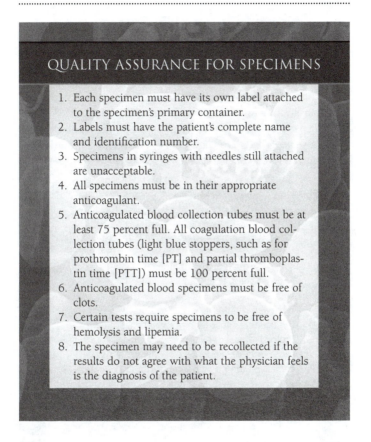

QUALITY ASSURANCE FOR SPECIMENS

1. Each specimen must have its own label attached to the specimen's primary container.
2. Labels must have the patient's complete name and identification number.
3. Specimens in syringes with needles still attached are unacceptable.
4. All specimens must be in their appropriate anticoagulant.
5. Anticoagulated blood collection tubes must be at least 75 percent full. All coagulation blood collection tubes (light blue stoppers, such as for prothrombin time [PT] and partial thromboplastin time [PTT]) must be 100 percent full.
6. Anticoagulated blood specimens must be free of clots.
7. Certain tests require specimens to be free of hemolysis and lipemia.
8. The specimen may need to be recollected if the results do not agree with what the physician feels is the diagnosis of the patient.

Factors Affecting Laboratory Values

Numerous variables can affect test results. The specimens are tested by analytical instruments that give accurate and precise results. These results only accurately reflect what is wrong with the patient if the sample is correctly collected. A correctly collected specimen is the responsibility of the phlebotomist. Patient physiological factors may also contribute to inaccurate results.

The patient can knowingly or unknowingly alter the results by certain actions. An example of this occurs when patients say they have had nothing to eat or drink, but they have had a cup of coffee. The patient is often under the misconception that black coffee without sugar is not a problem. Coffee and smoking affect the metabolism and so can alter test results.

FACTORS THAT CAN ALTER RESULTS

Patient-controlled factors that can alter test results include the following:

1. Fasting—If the patient is not in a fasting state when he or she should have been, results of tests will not be accurate. Glucose values will be elevated.
2. Prolonged fasting—Fasting for more than 14 hours causes increases and decreases in certain tests.
   Increases: amino acids, bilirubin, fatty acids, glucagon, growth hormone, ketones, lactate, triglycerides
   Decreases: glucose, high-density lipoprotein (HDL) cholesterol, insulin, lactate dehydrogenase (LDH), T3
3. Stress—Stress can have an effect. In children, violent crying before a specimen is collected raises the white blood cell (WBC) count up to 146 percent.
4. Exercise—Strenuous short-term exercise can make the heart work harder and increase the heart enzymes and WBC count.

Phlebotomist-controlled factors include the following:

1. Tourniquet—Hemoconcentration, a change in chemical concentration, which can result from a tourniquet tied too tightly, causes elevated levels of potassium, total protein, calcium, bilirubin, alanine aminotransferase (ALT), aspartate aminotransferase (AST), cholesterol, triglycerides, albumin, hemoglobin, and cell counts.

2. Heparin—Using an incorrect heparin tube can interfere with tests being run.

3. Correct volume—Not enough blood drawn causes a dilution that can change the size of the cells and therefore cause a variation in test results.

4. Inappropriate use of gel tubes—The gel can effect results of some therapeutic drug levels and blood bank testing.

5. Test exposed to light—Some tests must not be exposed to light. Vitamin E and bilirubin will have lower values after 1 hour of exposure to light. Amber tubes or foil-wrapped tubes will protect the specimen.

6. Incomplete sterilization of blood culture collection site—The incomplete sterilization of blood culture collection sites will result in a false positive blood culture. This causes a prolonged patient stay and increased cost to the patient.

7. Diurnal rhythm—Some specimens must be drawn at timed intervals because of medication or diurnal rhythm. The exact time of collection must also be noted on the specimen.

Chilling or Warming of Specimens

Certain specimens must be chilled or kept warmed immediately after collection. To chill a specimen, place the blood tube into an ice and water mixture as it is withdrawn from the evacuated tube holder (Figure 2.31). The mixture of ice and water provides an increased surface area to cool the specimen. This specimen should then be placed in a biohazard bag for transport. Make sure that the label will not come off in the water and the ink will not run, leaving the label

FIGURE 2.31 *Icing a specimen in ice and water solution.*

unreadable. If this is the case, label the tube, place the tube in a bag, and then place this tube in the ice and water mixture.

To keep a specimen warm, wrap an infant heel warmer around the specimen (Figure 2.32). Any delay in icing or warming the specimen will alter test results. The longer the delay, the greater the change. The phlebotomist must refer to the laboratory directory of service to determine if a specimen needs to be iced or warmed.

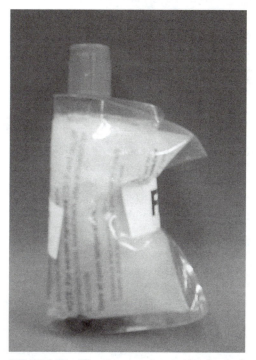

FIGURE 2.32 *Warming a specimen with infant heel warmer.*

Blood Cultures

Blood cultures are collected whenever it is suspected that a patient has septicemia. Septicemia is a condition in which microorganisms (mainly bacteria) circulate and multiply in the patient's blood. Because blood is normally sterile, the presence of microorganisms and their products is very serious and can result in death. The blood is collected and placed in a bottle that contains a solution that enhances the growth of significant microorganisms. An anticoagulant is also present. The microorganisms can then be cultured and identified so the most effective antibiotic treatment can be started.

If blood cultures are to be collected after antimicrobial treatment has started, the blood culture must be drawn in a special bottle containing a solution to inactivate the antimicrobial agent. This will then allow the bacteria to grow.

The volume of blood needed is critical to optimum recovery of the microorganisms. From 8 to 10 milliliters of blood is to be placed in the bottle. The optimum amount of blood varies depending on the manufacturer of the blood culture bottles. Adult draws need a total of 20 milliliters for the best recovery of microorganisms. Any lesser amount will reduce the recovery rate and lengthen the time to recovery. For infants and children, 1 to 4 milliliters of blood in a pediatric bottle is sufficient.

For adults, blood cultures are drawn in sets of two bottles. One bottle is the aerobic bottle for those microorganisms that need oxygen to grow. The second bottle is an anaerobic bottle for the microorganisms requiring an environment without oxygen. A set of blood cultures traditionally were collected at the height of the patient's fever. This is when the microorganisms were thought to be at their greatest number in the blood. With the new high-recovery blood culture bottles being used, drawing of the blood at the height of the fever is not as critical. Even during a low point of the fever, the microorganisms are present in sufficient number for rapid growth. Two blood culture sets are usually sufficient for recovery of significant microorganisms. These two sets consist of an aerobic and anaerobic blood culture collected from one patient site, such as the left arm, and another set of aerobic and anaerobic bottles collected from an alternate location. Ideally, the two sets are collected before starting antibiotic therapy.

The most critical step in collecting a blood culture is the proper cleaning of the site when doing a venipuncture. The site must be as clean as possible to avoid contaminating the blood culture with skin surface microorganisms and producing a false-positive blood culture. Commercial kits are available that can help with the cleaning (Figure 2.33).

FIGURE 2.33 *Skin cleaning kit for blood cultures.*

Procedure 2.6

BLOOD CULTURE COLLECTION

Principle:

To obtain venous blood acceptable for laboratory testing as required by a physician. Venous blood is collected by a butterfly needle system directly into blood culture containers.

Materials:

Gloves.

Goggles and mask.

Evacuated tube holder.

Butterfly needle system, 21- or 23-gauge needle with or without Leur adapter.

Syringe if not using Leur adapter on butterfly needle.

22-gauge syringe needle.

Tube holder for blood culture bottles.

Aerobic and anaerobic blood culture bottles.

Blood culture skin cleaning kit.

Tourniquet.

70 percent isopropyl alcohol swab.

Gauze or cotton balls.

Adhesive bandage or tape.

Sharps container.

Procedure:

1. Identify the patient. Inpatient: Verify identification bracelet name and hospital number with computer requisition information. Outpatient:

continues

Procedure 2.6 *continued*

BLOOD CULTURE COLLECTION

   Ask patient's name and verify with computer
   label or identification numbers.

2. Wash hands.

3. Don gloves. Putting on gloves may be delayed
   until step 12 for nonisolation patients.

4. Collect equipment.

5. Open the package of the butterfly needle system
   with evacuated tube Leur adapter. Thread the
   Leur needle into the special blood culture bottle
   holder (Figure 2.34).

6. The recommended fill for each blood culture bottle is 8 to 10 milliliters of blood. Mark each bottle

FIGURE 2.34 *Attaching butterfly to special blood culture bottle holder.*

continues

Procedure 2.6 *continued*

BLOOD CULTURE COLLECTION

8 to 10 milliliters above the level of the culture media using the scale on the side of the bottle.

7. Remove the plastic flip top or overcap from the aerobic and anaerobic bottles and disinfect the top of the bottles with an alcohol pad.

8. Apply the tourniquet.

9. Ask the patient to close the hand. The patient must not be allowed to pump the hand. If possible, place the patient's arm in a downward position.

10. Feel for a vein noting the location and direction of the vein.

11. Verify the patient is not allergic to iodine. Clean the venipuncture site using the special blood culture cleaning kit. Scrub with an alcohol scrub pad; allow the alcohol to dry, then clean with an iodine solution in a circular motion from the center outward. Allow sufficient time for the iodine to dry. The drying action helps kill the skin surface bacteria.

12. Don gloves if not done in step 3.

13. Do not touch the venipuncture site. If there is a potential for blood spatter, goggles and a mask must be worn.

14. Draw the skin taut with your thumb and index finger. Place the index finger at the point the vein was felt and the thumb 1 to 2 inches below the puncture site.

continues

Procedure 2.6 *continued*

BLOOD CULTURE COLLECTION

15. Hold the butterfly with the bevel up. With the bevel up, line up the needle with the vein and perform the venipuncture.

16. Do not enter the vein at the exact location at which the vein is felt. Enter the vein approximately ¼ inch below the vein location. The location where the vein was palpated is the point where the bevel of the needle must be in the vein. Push the needle into the skin. A sensation of resistance will be followed by easy penetration as the vein is entered. This is known as feeling the "pop." Once this point is reached, you should see a flash of blood in the needle tubing. Stop and do not move.

17. Remove your hand from drawing the skin taut. Grasp the tube holder and place it over the top of the aerobic blood culture bottle (Figure 2.35). Push the holder down to allow blood to enter the bottle. Remove the holder when the bottle volume reaches the previously marked line.

18. Fill the anaerobic bottle second. Due to air in the tubing, the aerobic bottle must be filled first to avoid contaminating the anaerobic bottle.

19. Ask the patient to open the hand.

20. Release the tourniquet.

21. Lightly place a gauze square or cotton ball above the venipuncture site.

22. Remove the needle from the arm.

continues

Procedure 2.6 *continued*

BLOOD CULTURE COLLECTION

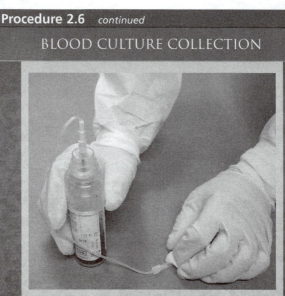

FIGURE 2.35 *Proper placement of holder on blood culture bottle.*

23. Activate the safety shield on the needle.

24. Apply pressure to the site for three to five minutes. The patient may assist if able. The arm should be elevated to reduce blood flow.

25. Dispose of the needle and holder in a sharps container. When disposing, insert the needle end of the device first and allow the tubing and holder to drop into the container.

26. Label bottles at the patient's side before leaving the examination room.

27. Apply an adhesive bandage.

Urine Collection

Procedures and standards for the collection of specimens other than blood are often ignored because the patient is doing the collection. Even more time should be spent discussing these procedures with the patient so the best possible specimen may be obtained. Without these instructions, the results will vary depending on how the patient collected the specimen. Residue from unclean containers (anything from butter tubs to soda bottles have been used by patients) can alter results dramatically. Patient cooperation is needed for any specimen to be accurate.

Urine is the most common specimen to collect besides blood. The laboratory should provide the container to ensure cleanliness of the specimen. For specimens that are to be used for a culture, the container must be sterile (Figure 2.36). The urine can consist of a cleancatch midstream random specimen, first morning specimen, timed specimen, or 24-hour specimen, to name a few.

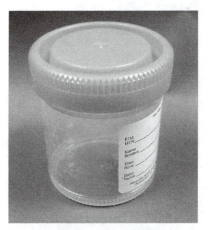

FIGURE 2.36 *Sterile urine collection container.*

If urine testing is delayed for more than an hour after collection, special precautions must be taken. Refrigeration of the specimen delays the deterioration of the specimen. An alternative to refrigeration is to transfer the urine into special urine evacuated tubes that contain preservative. A urine transfer straw is inserted into the urine cup and then the evacuated tubes are filled in the same manner as a blood evacuated tube (Figure 2.37).

The cleancatch midstream random specimen is collected at any time during a 24-hour period. The patient voids in a collection container at the time the specimen is needed. The patient cleans himself or herself, voids a little in the toilet, and then collects the urine specimen. The procedures are slightly different depending on whether the patient is a male or female (Procedures 2.7 and 2.8). The first morning specimen is collected in the same manner; it is just done when the patient first gets up in the morning.

FIGURE 2.37 *Urine preservative tubes and urine transfer straw.*

A 24-hour collection requires the most patient cooperation. The patient voids and discards the first morning specimen. All urine, including the next morning specimen, is then saved in a special container supplied by the laboratory (Figure 2.38). The patient must cooperate and not discard a single specimen (Procedure 2.9). Many 24-hour urine collections require that a preservative be placed into the container before collection. The patient must be notified about what the liquid in the container is and told not to pour it out.

FIGURE 2.38 *Twenty-four hour urine collection container with labels indicating acid has been added to container.*

Procedure 2.7

COLLECTING A CLEANCATCH MIDSTREAM URINE SPECIMEN: MALE

Principle:

To properly and safely collect a urine specimen from a male patient. The specimen is a cleancatch specimen taken from the midstream of the urine, collected in a sterile screw-top container.

Materials:

Gloves.

Hand disinfectant.

Sterile urine container.

Antiseptic wipes.

Label and requisition.

Procedure:

1. Wash hands carefully using soap and water.

2. Using one of the antiseptic wipes, cleanse the glans (tip) of the penis. If you are not circumcised, this is done while holding the foreskin back. Clean the area around the opening completely. Discard the wipe.

3. Following the first cleansing, wipe thoroughly using the second antiseptic wipe, while maintaining the foreskin in a retracted position. Discard the wipe.

4. Void a small amount of urine in the toilet bowl.

5. Continue to void and collect the urine in the cup. Do not touch the specimen cup on the inside or touch your body or clothing to the cup.

continues

Procedure 2.7 *continued*
COLLECTING A CLEANCATCH MIDSTREAM URINE SPECIMEN: MALE

6. Place the lid carefully onto the specimen container. Screw the lid on tightly to prevent leakage.
7. Give the urine to the phlebotomist.

Procedure 2.8
COLLECTING A CLEANCATCH MIDSTREAM URINE SPECIMEN: FEMALE

Principle:

To properly and safely collect a urine specimen from a female patient. The specimen is a cleancatch specimen taken from the midstream of the urine, collected in a sterile screw-top container.

Materials:

Gloves.

Hand disinfectant.

Sterile urine container.

Antiseptic wipes.

Label and requisition.

continues

Procedure 2.8 *continued*

COLLECTING A CLEANCATCH MIDSTREAM URINE SPECIMEN: FEMALE

Procedure:

1. Wash hands carefully using soap and water.

2. Remove underclothing.

3. Sit comfortably on the toilet seat and swing one knee to the side as far as you can.

4. Spread the labia with one hand and continue to keep them apart.

5. Clean the labia. Be sure to cleanse well before you collect the specimen.

   a. Using one of the antiseptic wipes, wipe from the front of your body toward the back. Clean between the folds of the skin as carefully as you can. Discard the wipe.

   b. Using the second antiseptic wipe, clean the area again using a front-to-back motion. Discard the wipe.

6. Pass a small amount of urine into the toilet bowl.

7. Continue to void and collect the urine in the cup. Do not touch the specimen cup on the inside or touch your body or clothing to the cup.

8. Place the lid carefully onto the specimen container. Screw the lid on tightly to prevent leakage.

9. Give the urine to the phlebotomist.

Procedure 2.9

COLLECTING A 24-HOUR URINE SPECIMEN

Principle:

To obtain a 24-hour urine collection, which is used to determine the 24-hour distribution of certain urine chemical output. Certain solutes exhibit diurnal variations, being higher or lower at different times of the 24-hour period. A complete 24-hour cycle shows the distribution of these variations in the total collection. Due to the length of time the urine must be collected, a preservative may need to be added before collection or refrigeration of the specimen may be necessary. The urine sample is collected in a 24-hour urine container and a preservative is added if necessary.

Materials:

Gloves.

Hand disinfectant.

24-hour urine container.

Antiseptic wipes.

Additives for urine preservative.

Label and requisition.

Procedure:

1. Obtain a 24-hour urine specimen container from the laboratory. Be careful not to touch or spill any additive that may have been placed in the container before collection.

continues

Procedure 2.9   *continued*

COLLECTING A 24-HOUR URINE SPECIMEN

2. Void and discard the first morning specimen, and record the time.

3. Collect all urine voided during the next 24 hours. Urine should be refrigerated or kept in a cool place throughout the collection period.

4. At exactly the same time the following morning, void completely and add this specimen to the container.

5. Deliver the specimen to the laboratory the morning the collection was stopped. The phlebotomist will ask your name, height, weight, and the time the test was started and stopped.

6. A blood sample may also need to be collected at this time.

U N I T

3

Microcollection

Sometimes the only alternative to collect a blood sample is to collect blood from the finger in adults or the heel in infants. Special equipment is needed to obtain accurate results when obtaining blood from the capillaries.

The type of specimen being collected limits this method. Certain tests require more blood than can be obtained from the capillaries.

Microcollection Equipment

Lancets

A lancet is a sterile, single-use, disposable, sharp-pointed instrument used to pierce the skin to obtain droplets of blood used for testing. Only lancets specifically designed for skin puncture should be used. To avoid penetrating bone, depth of puncture must be controlled.

A number of different skin puncture lancets are commercially available to puncture the skin for an adequate blood flow. This free flow of blood is the key to achieving an acceptable specimen. Surgical blades used in the past carried the hazard of puncturing too

FIGURE 3.1 *Non–spring-loaded lancets.*

deeply, especially with heelsticks in newborns or in pediatric patients. Lancets have now been designed for a controlled depth of puncture, and surgical blades should be used only for surgery. Lancets consist of either a blade the phlebotomist pushes into the skin (Figure 3.1) or a spring-loaded device (Figure 3.2) that makes the puncture to a prescribed depth. Apprehension of the puncture can be an obstacle the phlebotomist must overcome with the patient. Children can become so apprehensive that they pull their hand out of the caregiver's grasp just as the phlebotomist is ready to stick. The best device to use is the spring-loaded puncture device. These hide the blade in a plastic holder so the patient cannot see the blade doing the puncture. The plastic device lies on the skin, and the trigger is depressed. The spring forces the blade into the skin rapidly and then retracts. The rapid puncture and not seeing the blade leaves the patient less apprehensive to skin punctures. The spring-loaded blades work by a guillotine action or a

FIGURE 3.2 *Spring-loaded puncture devices.*

slicing motion. Devices can be purchased that puncture no more than 2 millimeters for newborn heelsticks. Other devices vary in depth for fingersticks of different-age patients. What should be avoided when collecting samples for laboratory specimens are the devices on the market for diabetic at-home blood glucose monitoring. These devices are excellent for their purpose but do not provide a blood flow of more than one or two drops. This is not adequate for the sample size needed for most laboratory testing.

Capillary Tubes and Microcollection Devices

The devices used for collecting, processing, and transporting microcollections depend on the laboratory testing being performed. Disposable capillary micropipettes are thin-bore devices much like small soda straws that draw the blood up to a certain line on the tubing. The line on the tubing indicates the calibration for an amount drawn from 1 to 200 microliters. They are generally used for measurement of an amount of blood and then transferred to a container or solution. The blood draws up into the tube because of capillary action. The capillary action of a tube is enhanced if the tube is slanted in a semihorizontal direction as the blood is being drawn into the tube. Plastic or plastic coating has replaced glass for the micropipettes due to the safety hazard of broken glass.

Microhematocrit capillary tubes are narrow-bore pipettes primarily intended for determining packed red cell volume in microsamples. Once filled, the tubes are centrifuged in a special centrifuge that packs the formed elements of the blood. This packed volume is then read on a scale that gives the packed volume as a percentage of the total. The result is the hematocrit of the patient. Because the volume is read on a special sliding scale, the total volume in the tube is not important. The volume required for the tube is 50 to 75 microliters.

Blood gas collection pipettes collect skin puncture whole blood specimens under anaerobic conditions for blood gas determinations. The tubes vary in size but draw 50 to 250 microliters of volume. The size of the draw needed depends on the instrument used in the blood gas testing. The tubes contain heparin to keep the blood from clotting and can be plugged with sealant putty or caps to maintain anaerobic conditions.

The process of collection and transfer of blood samples has been simplified with the use of plastic microcollection devices. These devices consist of small nonsterile plastic containers. They have included a means for filling, measuring, color-coding for the proper anticoagulant, stoppering, centrifugation, and storage. The color coding matches the coding on the anticoagulant

FIGURE 3.3 *Microcollection devices.*

tubes: lavender is EDTA, green is heparin, and red gives a serum sample. The serum tubes can contain the thixotropic separator gel that separates the serum from the cells after centrifugation. Bilirubin samples are collected in an amber tube that protects the blood from light. If a bilirubin specimen is not protected from light, the bilirubin level of the blood in the tube will rapidly decrease.

Accurate test results require all microcollection specimens to be collected with a free-flowing sample. As the drop of blood forms, the collection cap, which consists of a scoop or tubing device in the cap, touches it. The blood then flows into the bottom of the tube. The tubes hold approximately 600 microliters of blood. They go by a variety of brand names, such as Microtainer and Microvette (Figure 3.3).

Skin Puncture Blood Collection

Blood is not taken in large amounts at once from the fingerstick. It is taken in small amounts through the capillary blood flow. Blood flowing away from the heart flows in the arteries. Blood flowing back to the heart flows in the veins. Connecting most of the arteries and veins are the capillaries. Due to the one-way blood flow, the composition of the blood released from the capillary area during skin puncture is primarily arterial blood.

The artery has a thick wall that helps it withstand the pressure of the pumping of the heart. The arteries branch to form arterioles that branch more to become capillaries. The capillaries then start

FIGURE 3.4 *Infant heel warmer.*

converging to form venules, and the venules then become veins. As blood flows through the body, it follows this path of artery-capillary-vein. Oxygenated arterial blood leaves the heart and carries this oxygen to the tissue by releasing the oxygen through the cell walls of the capillaries. At the same time, carbon dioxide is being absorbed by the blood and then transported to the lungs to be exhaled as a waste product. The flow of the blood also regulates body temperature. When the body gets warm, the capillaries in the extremities dilate (enlarge in diameter) and let off heat. This process then cools the body. If the body becomes cold, the capillaries constrict (get smaller in diameter) and less blood flows through, thereby conserving heat for the rest of the body. This can be used to an advantage when collecting blood from the capillaries. Warming the site to 42°C for three minutes increases the blood flow by seven times. Warming can be done by using a warm washcloth, having the patient hold the hands under warm running water, or using an infant heel warmer (Figure 3.4).

Obtaining a Blood Sample from a Fingerstick

The skin puncture is the method of choice in children under one year old and for adults whose veins are inaccessible. Skin puncture is done by puncturing the skin. As the patient bleeds, the blood is collected in the appropriate microcollection equipment. Adult skin punctures are done in the finger; with children under one year old, the foot is the puncture site of choice.

Patients who are severely dehydrated or have poor circulation (those in shock, for example) cannot produce a skin puncture blood sample. A patient who is extremely cold also will not produce adequate blood flow. This last situation can be rectified by warming the hand.

The site for the collection of a skin puncture in an adult is on the palmar surface of the distal phalanx of the finger. The side or tip of the finger should not be punctured because the tissue is about half as thick as the tissue in the center of the finger. The fingers of choice are the middle finger and the ring finger (second and third fingers). The puncture site must be warm or have been warmed, and the finger must not be swollen from the buildup of fluids (edematous). Puncturing an edematous finger contaminates the sample with the tissue fluid. When you puncture the finger, cut across the fingerprint line. This technique delivers the best possible blood flow and facilitates the formation of drops of blood. If the cut is made between the fingerprint lines, the fingerprints exert a pressure on the cut and close the cut. The blood follows the lines of the fingerprint, resulting in no droplet formation.

Clean the finger with isopropanol (alcohol) and then dry with sterile gauze or allow to air dry thoroughly before any puncture. If the alcohol is not dry and contaminates the blood sample, the sample will become hemolyzed. Do not use povidone-iodine (Betadine) to clean and disinfect the puncture site. Even if Betadine has been allowed to thoroughly dry, it will cause elevated potassium, phosphorous, and uric acid levels.

Think before the puncture. As you hold the patient's hand, the underside of the finger may need to be the side punctured. After the puncture, the blood drips downward and gravity helps the blood flow into the collector. Before the blood sample is collected, the first drop of blood needs to be wiped away. As the finger is punctured, tissue cells are damaged, and interstitial fluid is released into the first drop. The subsequent drops are flowing due to arterial pressure.

If the puncture is adequate, 0.5 milliliters of blood can be collected from a single puncture. As the drop of blood forms at the puncture site, touch the tip of the microcollection device to the drop. Blood flow can be further enhanced by gently applying continuous pres-

CAUSES OF HEMOLYSIS IN CAPILLARY PUNCTURE

1. The alcohol used to clean the skin was not allowed to dry.
2. The finger or heel was squeezed too hard to produce a greater blood flow.
3. The specimen was taken from a newborn. Newborn infants have increased red blood cell fragility and a high red blood cell volume. These factors result in a greater amount of hemolysis.
4. Instead of allowing the blood to flow into the microcollection container, the blood was scrapped off the skin surface

sure to the surrounding tissue. Rapid milking of the finger does not enhance the blood flow. Excess pressure may cause hemolysis or contamination of the specimen with tissue fluid.

Several problems can cause inaccurate test results. Hemolysis is the greatest concern with microcollection samples.

Hemolysis as measured by the concentration of free hemoglobin due to ruptured red blood cells in the serum or plasma of the blood may not be readily apparent. This is particularly so in the case of those newborns with elevated bilirubin levels. The yellow of the serum may mask the red hemolysis.

Producing a specimen without clots is also a challenge in microcollection. The body turns on its defenses to clot the blood at the puncture site and stop the bleeding as soon as the skin is punctured. These defenses create problems when a whole blood sample is needed. If an EDTA specimen is required, that specimen is drawn first to obtain an adequate volume before the blood starts to clot and platelet clumping occurs. Any other additive specimens are collected next, with clotted specimens last. If the blood has started to produce microscopic clots while filling the last tube, there is not a problem because the blood is going to be allowed to clot in the tube.

ORDER OF DRAW FOR FINGERSTICK SAMPLE COLLECTION

1. Capillary blood gases
2. Blood smears
3. EDTA microcontainers (mix well after collection)
4. Other additive microcontainers (mix well after collection)
5. Nonadditive microcontainers (clot tubes)
6. Metabolic screen cards

Procedure 3.1

CAPILLARY BLOOD COLLECTION

Principle:

To obtain capillary blood acceptable for laboratory testing as requested by a physician. The volume collected is dependent upon the test(s) ordered.

continues

Procedure 3.1 *continued*

CAPILLARY BLOOD COLLECTION

Materials:

Disposable sterile lancet.

Sterile gauze squares or cotton balls.

Alcohol swabs.

Gloves.

Sharps container.

Collection containers as required by test(s).

Capillary tubes.

Diluting fluids.

Calibrated pipettes.

Microcollection containers.

Glass slides.

Filter paper for metabolic screen.

Procedure:

1. Identify the patient. Inpatient: Verify identification bracelet name and hospital number with computer requisition information. Outpatient: Ask the patient's name and verify with computer label or identification numbers.

2. If a fasting specimen is required, ask the patient when he or she last ate. Explain the procedure to the patient.

3. Wash hands.

4. Don gloves.

continues

Procedure 3.1 *continued*

CAPILLARY BLOOD COLLECTION

5. Assemble equipment. Select the appropriate puncture device. Select the appropriate containers for blood collection. Place the equipment within easy reach, and make any necessary preparation of fluids or containers.

6. Select the puncture site. Warm if necessary using a heel warmer or warm washcloth for three minutes.

7. Finger: Use the central fleshy area of the third or fourth fingers (palmar surface of the distal phalanx of the finger).

8. Heel: Use the fleshy area at the side curvature of the heel (the most medial or lateral portion of the plantar surface).

9. Choose the finger for the puncture site that is not cold or edematous.

10. If all fingers are cold, warm the hand three minutes with a warm washcloth.

11. Gently massage the finger using a milking action to increase blood flow potential (Figure 3.5).

12. Clean the puncture site with 70 percent isopropyl alcohol and let the area dry.

13. Place the puncture device firmly on the puncture site (Figure 3.6).

14. Fingerstick: The blade should be aligned to cut across the grooves of the fingerprint.

continues

Procedure 3.1 *continued*

CAPILLARY BLOOD COLLECTION

15. Heel: Place the blade spot of the lancet against the heel so its center point is vertically aligned with the desired incision site.

16. Puncture the skin with the disposable lancet.

17. Wipe away the first drop of blood with a sterile dry gauze or cotton ball (Figure 3.7)

18. Collect the specimen in the chosen container (Figure 3.8). Touch only the tip of the collection tube to the drop of blood. Blood flow is en-

FIGURE 3.5 *Massage the finger to increase the flow of blood.*

FIGURE 3.6 *Place the puncture device firmly on the puncture site.*

FIGURE 3.7 *Wipe away the first drop of blood.*

FIGURE 3.8 *Collect the specimen in the chosen container.*

continues

Procedure 3.1 *continued*

CAPILLARY BLOOD COLLECTION

couraged if the puncture site is held in a downward angle and a gentle pressure applied to the finger. The order of collection is as follows:

a. Capillary blood gases.

b. Blood smears.

c. EDTA microcontainers (mix well after collection).

d. Other additive microcontainers (mix well after collection).

e. Nonadditive microcontainers (clot tubes).

f. Metabolic screen card.

19. Seal the specimen containers.

20. Apply pressure to the puncture site with a gauze square or cotton ball.

21. Label the collection containers.

22. If an insufficient sample has been obtained, the puncture may be repeated at a different site. A new sterile lancet and new collection containers must be used.

REFERENCES

Centers for Disease Control and Prevention, National Institute for Occupational Safety and Health, U.S. Department of Health and Human Service, Public Health Service. *Preventing needlestick injuries in health care settings.* www.cdc.gov/niosh, or by calling 1-800-35-NIOSH.

Federal register, rules and regulations, 29 CFR Part 1910.1030. (1991, December 6). Vol. 56 (235).

Geller, S. J. (1992, March 3). *Effect of sample collection on laboratory test results.* ASCP Teleconference Series.

Hoeltke, L. B. (1995). *The clinical laboratory manual series: phlebotomy.* Albany, NY, Delmar.

Hoeltke, L. B. (2006). *The complete textbook of phlebotomy* (3rd ed.). Albany, NY, Delmar.

National Committee for Clinical Laboratory Standards. (1999). *Procedures and devices for the collection of diagnostic blood specimens by skin puncture* (4th ed.). Approved Standard. NCCLS Document H4-A4.Wayne, PA: Author.

National Committee for Clinical Laboratory Standards. (2002, December). *Protection of laboratory workers from occupationally acquired infections* (2nd ed.). Approved Standard. NCCLS Document M29-A2. Wayne, PA: Author.

National Committee for Clinical Laboratory Standards. (2003, December). *Procedures for the collection of diagnostic blood specimens by venipuncture* (5th ed.). Approved Standard. NCCLS Document H3-A5.Wayne, PA: Author.

National Committee for Clinical Laboratory Standards. (2003, December). *Tubes and additives for venous blood specimen collection* (5th ed.). Approved Standard. NCCLS Document H1-A5.Wayne, PA: Author.

Occupational Safety and Health Administration. (2001, April). *Revision to OSHA's bloodborne pathogens standard technical background and summary.* www.osha.gov/needlesticks/needefact.html.

APPENDIX

Phlebotomy Competency Assessment

(Example of observed competency check-off)

Student/Associate: _____

Venipuncture Collection with an Evacuated Tube System

Competency: Demonstrate proper patient identification and specimen collection technique when performing a venipuncture with an evacuated tube system.

Behavior: Identifies patient.

Uses appropriate collection tubes.

Follows correct collection procedure.

Follows order of draw.

#	Task	Satisfactory Performance 2 points	Improvement Needed 1 point	Unsatisfactory Performance 0 points
1	Identifies self and patient correctly.			
2	Checks requisition for all pertinent information.			
3	Washes hands.			
4	Explains procedure to patient.			
5	Selects correct tubes and equipment for procedure.			
6	Assembles equipment.			
7	Positions patient's arm.			
8	Ties tourniquet.			
9	Locates vein by palpation.			
10	Releases tourniquet if needed.			
11	Cleanses site in concentric circles and allows to air dry.			
12	Puts on gloves.			
13	Reapplies tourniquet if removed in step 10.			

#	Task	Satisfactory Performance 2 points	Improvement Needed 1 point	Unsatisfactory Performance 0 points
14	Positions needle holder between thumb and index finger.			
15	Uncaps needle. Inspects needle for defects.			
16	Anchors the vein.			
17	Positions needle at appropriate angle.			
18	Inserts needle bevel up into vein.			
19	Collects blood following order of draw			
20	Changes tubes smoothly; does not move needle.			
21	Releases tourniquet.			
22	Removes last tube collected from the holder.			
23	Covers puncture site with gauze or cotton ball.			
24	Withdraws needle smoothly and presses down on gauze or cotton.			

#	Task	Satisfactory Performance 2 points	Improvement Needed 1 point	Unsatisfactory Performance 0 points
25	Activates safety device on needle.			
26	Disposes of needle and holder in sharps container.			
27	Inverts tube(s) with additives several times.			
28	Labels specimen with correct draw time.			
29	Checks puncture site when procedure is complete.			
30	Disposes of used supplies in proper containers.			
31	Removes gloves and washes hands.			
32	Thanks and releases patient.			
	Total points in each category:			
	Total in all categories:			

Student/associate signature:

_____ Date: _____

Instructor signature:

_____ Date: _____

Supervisor signature:

_____ Date: _____

APPENDIX B

Phlebotomy Test Questions

Multiple Choice Questions

1. The gauge of the needle indicates the following relationship—the larger the gauge number, the:

   a. larger the diameter of the bore

   b. longer the needle

   c. shorter the needle

   d. smaller the diameter of the bore

2. If the blood is drawn too quickly from a vein, the vein will have a tendency to:

   a. bruise

   b. collapse

   c. disintegrate

   d. roll

3. The bevel of the needle:

   a. attaches to the syringe or the holder

   b. should be held at a 50-degree angle to the skin

   c. should always be facing up when inserted into the skin

   d. should always be facing down when inserted into the skin

4. In which of the following conditions would you avoid a site for venipuncture?

   a. edematous arm

   b. arm with IV

   c. hematoma

   d. all of the above

5. In drawing blood samples, which of the following should be performed first?

   a. Clean the site.

   b. Find the vein.

   c. Apply the tourniquet.

   d. Identify the patient.

6. What is the major drawback of a 24-hour urine collection?

   a. The tests done are unreliable.

   b. Preservatives must be used.

   c. Doctors don't know when to order it.

   d. Patient cooperation is essential and often hard to get.

7. The components of blood found inside of a tube drawn with anticoagulant are:

   a. plasma, buffy coat, and erythrocytes

   b. buffy coat and clot

    c. serum and buffy coat

    d. serum and clot

8. Venipuncture is usually performed in the anticubital area. Which vein is *usually* the best to draw from?

    a. cephalic

    b. basilic

    c. median cubital

    d. none of the above

9. The gray-stoppered tube is usually drawn for which test?

    a. glucose

    b. PTT

    c. enzyme

    d. hematology

10. The doctor orders a CBC (lavender stopper), comprehensive metabolic panel (SST), PT (light blue stopper), and a set of blood cultures. What is the order of draw?

    a. SST tube, light blue, blood culture, lavender

    b. blood culture, light blue, lavender, SST

    c. blood culture, light blue, SST, lavender

    d. blood culture, green, light blue, SST

11. What can happen if the tourniquet is left on too long before drawing blood?

    a. hematoma

    b. hemolysis

    c. hemoconcentration

    d. none of the above

12. The formed elements make up about _____ percent of the whole blood volume.

    a. 30 percent

    b. 45 percent

    c. 55 percent

    d. 60 percent

13. All of the following statements are true EXCEPT:

    a. Gray-stoppered tubes are used for blood glucose tests.

    b. Gray-stoppered tubes are used for CBC and WBC tests.

    c. Lavender-stoppered tubes are used for CBC, WBC, and platelet testing.

    d. Red-stoppered tubes are used for many tests, including serum enzyme testing.

14. The depth of cut made by a lancet for a heelstick should be NO MORE THAN:

    a. 1.5 millimeters

    b. 2.0 millimeters

    c. 2.8 millimeters

    d. 3.0 millimeters

15. The single most important way to prevent the spread of infection in a hospital or other health care facility is:

    a. gowning and gloving

    b. handwashing

    c. always wearing gloves

    d. avoiding breathing on patients

16. The tourniquet should not be left on more than _____ minute(s) before a flow of blood is obtained.

    a. one

    b. four

    c. six

    d. ten

17. As a general rule, you should not stick a person more than _____ in an attempt to obtain blood.

    a. once

    b. twice

    c. three times

    d. four times

18. What is the best specimen for urine collection?

    a. any random specimen

    b. a catheterized specimen

    c. a cleancatch midstream urine specimen

    d. a specimen from an ostomy bag

19. The most common cause of blood culture contamination is:

    a. collection of too much blood

    b. collection of the sample from below the IV

    c. improper skin preparation

    d. use of a needle and syringe for collection

20. Serum is described as hemolyzed in the presence of:

    a. increased bilirubin causing jaundice

    b. increased carbon dioxide from cell metabolism

    c. increased hemoglobin due to ruptured RBCs

    d. increased lipids in a nonfasting sample

21. Why must the first drop of blood from a capillary puncture be wiped away?

    a. to remove interstitial (tissue) fluid

    b. to wipe away any bacterial contamination

    c. to remove heparin/saline contamination

    d. to make the blood flow faster

22. The following items are minimum requirements for specimen labeling:

    a. patient's complete name, identification number, date, time of collection, and physician

    b. patient's complete name, identification number, date, time of collection, and collector's initials

    c. patient's complete name and identification number

    d. patient's complete name, date, and time of collection

23. When serum is needed for testing, blood should be collected in which color stoppered tube?

    a. light blue

    b. green

    c. lavender

    d. red

24. The anticoagulant preferred for hematology testing is:

    a. citrate

    b. EDTA

    c. fluoride

    d. heparin

Matching Questions

25. _____ Contains no additive
26. _____ Contains glycolytic inhibitor (prevents glycolysis)
27. _____ Preserves the cell morphology for a differential
28. _____ Contains EDTA
29. _____ Requires a 1:9 ratio
30. _____ Contains a clot activator
31. _____ Contains heparin
32. _____ Contains oxalate
33. _____ Contains thixotropic gel
34. _____ Gives a serum sample (two answers)
35. _____ Gives a serum sample (two answers)

    a. glass red-stoppered tube

    b. light blue–stoppered tube

    c. green-stoppered tube

    d. lavender-stoppered tube

    e. gray-stoppered tube

    f. plastic SST tube

Critical Thinking Questions

1. Explain the difference between serum and plasma tubes. Find tubes in the laboratory that represent each type of tube.

2. A patient indicates he has a latex allergy. Explain the changes in equipment you would need to make to accommodate this patient.

3. You draw two light blue–stoppered tubes on a patient and both tubes fill only half full. What would be the problem if you poured the two tubes together to make a full tube, as you know is required with a light blue–stoppered tube?

4. Explain the difference between a glass red-stoppered tube and a plastic red-stoppered tube in the ability of the tube to clot.

5. The patient has an IV running in her right hand. The left arm is in a cast, so you go to the only available site, in the median cubital vein of the right arm, to collect your blood sample. The IV is running a saline solution, and you are going to collect a sample for glucose testing. You assume there will not be a problem. Are you correct?

Answers to Questions

1. d
2. b
3. c
4. d
5. d
6. d
7. a
8. c
9. a
10. c
11. c
12. b
13. b
14. b
15. b

16. a
17. b
18. c
19. c
20. c
21. a
22. b
23. d
24. b
25. a
26. e
27. d
28. d
29. b
30. f
31. c
32. e
33. f
34. a
35. f

Answers to Critical Thinking Questions

1. Serum tubes are tubes that are going to allow the blood within the tube to clot, therefore after centrifugation the liquid portion will be serum. A plasma tube has an anticoagulant chemical in the tube to prevent the blood from clotting. The liquid portion from this tube is plasma.

....

Some examples of serum tube are: red-stoppered, gold-stoppered, red/black stoppered. Examples of plasma tubes are: light blue-stoppered, lavender-stoppered, gray-stoppered, green-stoppered.

2. If a patient indicates they have a latex allergy you will need to clean the area that the patient will have contact with such as the chair and arm of the drawing chair. Wash your hands and use a latex free tourniquet, latex free gloves and latex free bandages.

3. The light blue-stoppered tube must be full with the proper blood to anticoagulant ratio. By pouring the two half filled tubes together you are doubling the anticoagulant and offsetting the proper ratio.

4. Both a glass and plastic red-stoppered tube will clot the blood. The plastic red-stoppered tube needs the have a clot activator within the tube in order for the tube to clot.

5. Collecting blood from the arm that has a saline IV running will dilute the blood sample with saline solution. This will give an inaccurate result for the glucose test.

INDEX

A

A, solution, 22
Allergy, latex, 51–52
Answers to questions, 134–135
Anticoagulants, 18–26
  gel separators, 24–26
  glass red-stoppered tubes, 23–24
  gray-stoppered tubes, 18–20
  green-stoppered tubes, 21–22
  lavender-stoppered tubes, 21
  light blue-stoppered tubes, 20
  orange-stoppered tubes, 22–23
  pink-stoppered tubes, 22
  plastic red-stoppered tubes, 24
  royal blue-stoppered tubes, 23
  sodium polyanthol sulfonate
    (SPS), 22
  solution A, 22
  solution B, 22
  white-stoppered tubes, 23

B

B, solution, 22
Blood
  icteric, 48–49
  lipemic, 49
Blood-borne pathogens, 5
Blood cells
  red, 14
  white, 14

Blood collection equipment,
    29–36
  butterfly, 34–36
  evacuated system, 32–34
  syringe system, 30–31
Blood collection, precautions in,
    47–49
  hematoma, 47–48
  hemoconcentration, 47
  hemolysis, 48
  icteric blood, 48–49
  lipemic blood, 49
Blood collection, skin puncture,
    112–113
Blood components, 14–18
Blood cultures, 92–98
Blood samples, collecting
    venipuncture, 53–86
  butterfly collection system,
    72–85
  evacuated tube specimen
    collection, 72
  positioning patients, 53
  selecting appropriate
    venipuncture sites, 54–55
  syringe specimen collection,
    63–72
  unsuccessful venipuncture,
    85–86
  vein stimulation, 56–62

Blood samples, obtaining from
    fingersticks, 113–120
Blue-stopped tubes
    light, 20
    royal, 23
Body substance isolation (BSI), 5
Butterfly system, 34–36, 72–85

C

Capillary tubes, 109–111
Cells
    red blood, 14
    white blood, 14
Cleaning of draw site, 38
Collection
    evacuated tube specimen, 72
    skin puncture blood, 112–113
    syringe specimen, 63–72
    urine, 99–106
Collection, precautions in blood,
    47–49
    hematoma, 47–48
    hemoconcentration, 47
    hemolysis, 48
    icteric blood, 48–49
    lipemic blood, 49
Collection system, butterfly, 72–85
Competency assessment, phlebotomy
    venipuncture collection with
    evacuated tube system,
    123–126
Components, blood, 14–18
Critical thinking questions,
    133–134
Cultures, blood, 92–98
Customer service, 3–4

D

Devices, microcollection, 109–111
Disinfecting, handwashing and,
    6–10

Draw site, cleaning of, 38
Drawing tubes, order of, 38–40

E

Equipment, blood collection, 29–36
    butterfly, 34–36
    evacuated system, 32–34
    syringe system, 30–31
Equipment, microcollection,
    107–111
    capillary tubes, 109–111
    lancets, 107–109
    microcollection devices,
    109–111
Erythrocytes, 14
Evacuated system, 32–34
Evacuated tube specimen
    collection, 72
Evacuated tube system,
    venipuncture collection
    with, 123–126

F

Fingersticks, obtaining blood
    samples from, 113–120
Forms, test request, 46 –47

G

Gel separators, 24–26
Glass red-stopped tubes, 23–24
Gloves, 10–14
Gray-stopped tubes, 18–20
Green-stopped tubes, 21–22

H

Handwashing, 51
    and disinfecting, 6–10
Hematoma, 47–48
Hemoconcentration, 47
Hemolysis, 48
Heparin/saline well, 50

I

Icteric blood, 48–49
Indwelling line, 50
Intravenous (IV) lines, 49–50

L

Labeling, specimen, 41–46
Laboratory values, factors affecting, 87–89
Lancets, 107–109
Latex allergy, 51–52
Lavender-stoppered tubes, 21
Leukocytes, 14
Light blue-stoppered tubes, 20
Lines
    indwelling, 50
    intravenous (IV), 49–50

M

Matching questions, 133–134
Microcollection, 107–120
    devices, 109–111
    equipment, 107–111
    obtaining blood samples from fingersticks, 113–120
    skin puncture blood collection, 112–113
Microcollection equipment, 107–111
    capillary tubes, 109–111
    lancets, 107–109
    microcollection devices, 109–111
Multiple choice questions, 127–132

N

Needle safety, 36–37

O

Orange-stoppered tubes, 22–23

P

Pathogens, blood-borne, 5
Patient satisfaction, 4–5
Patients, positioning, 53
Phlebotomy competency assessment, 123–126
Phlebotomy test questions, 127–135
    answers to questions, 134–135
    critical thinking questions, 133–134
    matching questions, 133
    multiple choice questions, 127–132
Pink-stoppered tubes, 22
Plastic red-stoppered tubes, 24
Platelets, 14
Precautions
    standard, 5
    universal, 5
Principles, venipuncture, 1–40
Puncture, skin, 112–113

Q

Questions, phlebotomy test, 127–135
    answers to questions, 134–135
    critical thinking questions, 133–134
    matching questions, 133–134
    multiple choice questions, 127–132

R

Red blood cells, 14
Red-stoppered tubes
    glass, 23–24
    plastic, 24
References, 121
Royal blue-stoppered tubes, 23

S

Safety, needle, 36–37
Saline well. *See* Heparin/saline well
Samples, collecting venipuncture
    blood, 53–86
    butterfly collection system,
        72–85
    evacuated tube specimen
        collection, 72
    positioning patients, 53
    selecting appropriate
        venipuncture sites, 54–55
    syringe specimen collection,
        63–72
    unsuccessful venipuncture,
        85–86
    vein stimulation, 56–62
Satisfaction, patient, 4–5
Separators, gel, 24–26
Service, customer, 3–4
Sites
    cleaning of draw, 38
    selecting appropriate
        venipuncture, 54–55
Skin puncture blood collection,
    112–113
Sodium polyanthol sulfonate (SPS),
    22
Solution A or B, 22
Specimen collection
    evacuated tube, 72
    syringe, 63–72
Specimen labeling, 41–46
Specimens
    chilling or warming of, 90–91
    re-collection or rejection of,
        86–87
Standard precautions, 5
Syringe specimen collection, 63–72
Syringe system, 30–31

System
    butterfly, 34–36, 72–85
    evacuated, 32–34
    syringe, 30–31
    Vacutainer, 32
    venipuncture collection with
        evacuated tube, 123–126

T

Technique, venipuncture, 41–106
Test questions, phlebotomy,
    127–135
    answers to questions, 134–135
    critical thinking questions,
        133–134
    matching questions, 133
    multiple choice questions,
        127–132
Test request form, 46–47
Thrombocytes, 14
Tourniquets, 56, 57
Tube system, venipuncture
        collection with evacuated,
        123–126
Tubes
    capillary, 109–111
    glass red-stoppered, 23–24
    gray-stoppered, 18–20
    green-stoppered, 21–22
    lavender-stoppered, 21
    light blue-stoppered, 20
    many choices in types of tubes,
        26–29
    orange-stoppered, 22–23
    order of drawing, 38–40
    pink-stoppered, 22
    plastic red-stoppered, 24
    royal blue-stoppered, 23
    white-stoppered, 23

U

Universal precautions, 5
Unsuccessful venipuncture, 85–86
Urine collection, 99–106

V

Vacutainer system, 32
Vascular access device (VAD),
    50–51
Vein stimulation, 56–62
Venipuncture blood samples,
    collecting, 53–86
    butterfly collection system,
        72–85
    evacuated tube specimen
        collection, 72
    positioning patients, 53
    selecting appropriate
        venipuncture sites, 54–55
    syringe specimen collection,
        63–72
    unsuccessful venipuncture,
        85–86
    vein stimulation, 56–62
Venipuncture collection with
    evacuated tube system,
    123–126
Venipuncture principles, 1–40
    anticoagulants, 18–26
    blood collection equipment,
        29–36
    blood components, 14–18
    cleaning of draw site, 38
    customer service, 3–4
    focusing on patients, 1–3

many choices in types of tubes,
    26–29
needle safety, 36–37
order of drawing tubes, 38–40
patient satisfaction, 4–5
standard precaution, 5–14
Venipuncture sites, selecting
    appropriate, 54–55
Venipuncture technique, 41–106
    blood cultures, 92–98
    chilling or warming of
        specimens, 90–91
    collecting venipuncture blood
        samples, 53–86
    factors affecting laboratory
        values, 87–89
    handwashing, 51
    intravenous (IV) lines, 49–50
    latex allergy, 51–52
    precautions in blood collection,
        46–47
    re-collection or rejection of
        specimens, 86–87
    specimen labeling, 41–46
    test request form, 46–47
    urine collection, 99–106
    vascular access device (VAD),
        50–51
Venipuncture, unsuccessful, 85–86

W

Well, heparin/saline, 50
White blood cells, 14
White-stopped tubes, 23